Dementia Day by Day

Dementia Day by Day

A Caretaker's Diary

David Legan

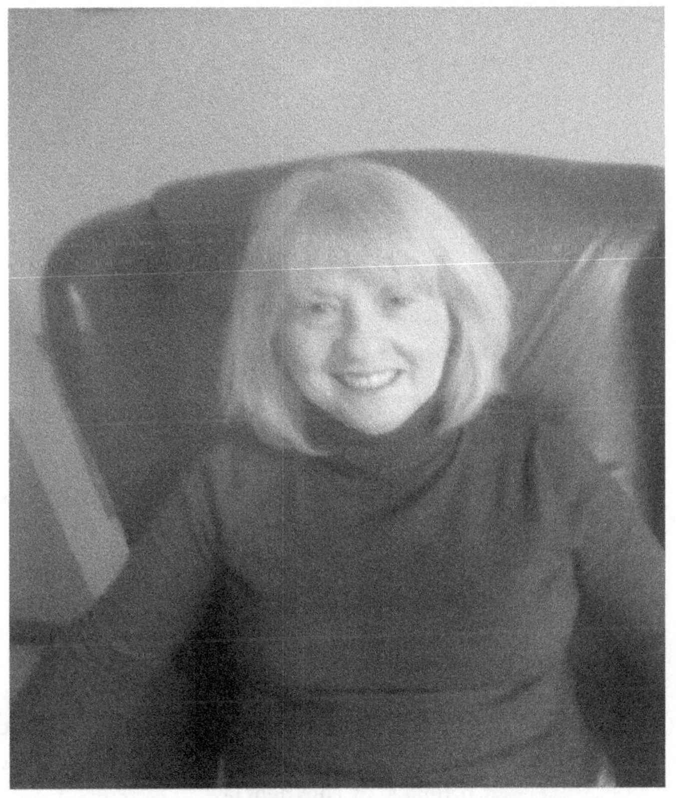

Shannon Woodruff, 2019

David Legan
Dementia Day by Day

Published by Spines
ISBN 979-8-89569-962-1

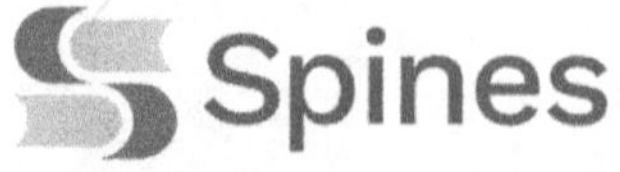

Contents

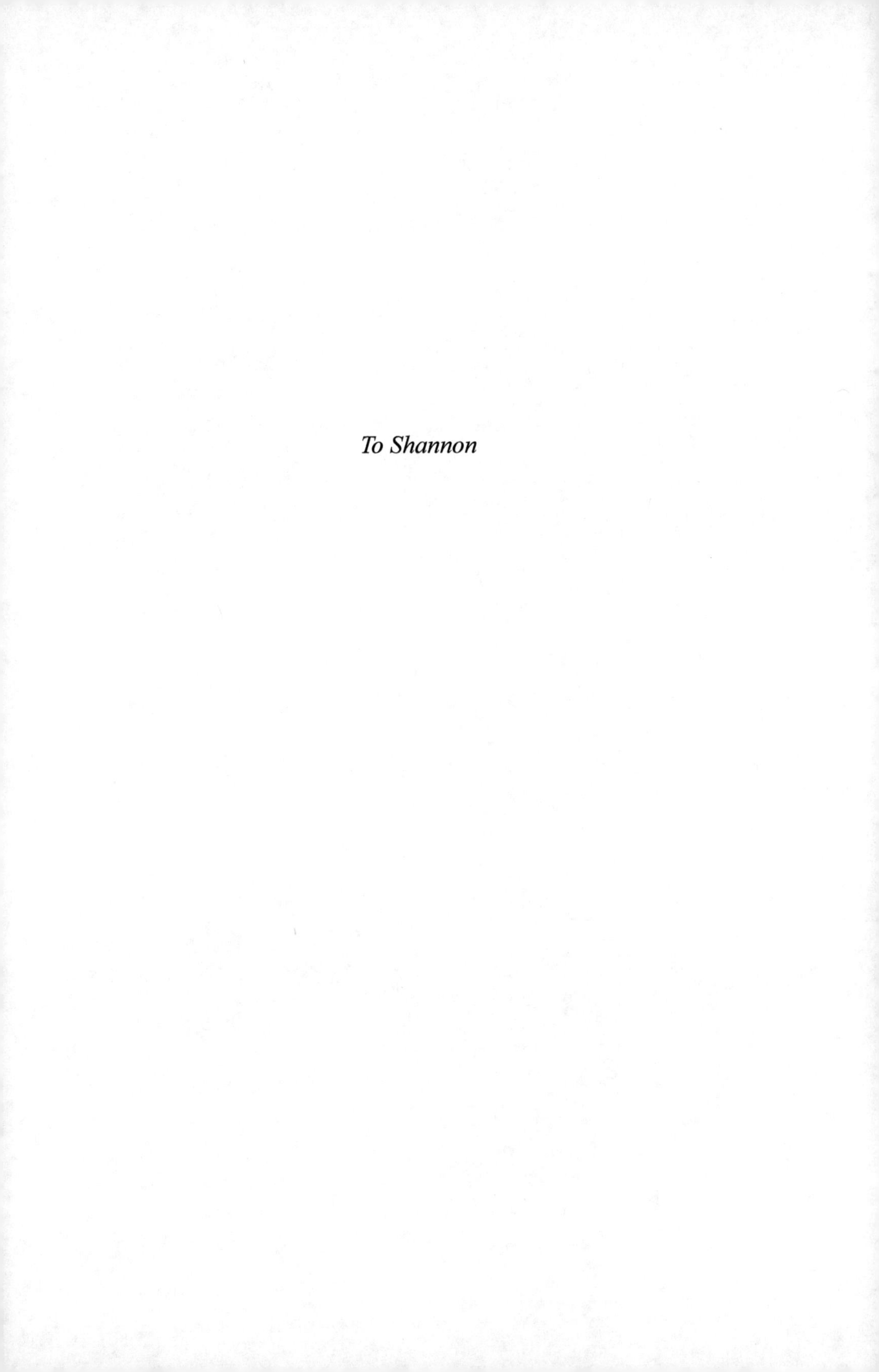

To Shannon

Foreword

She told him not to worry, said he'd be fine when she was gone.
Sam Baker

"Shannon's Story" was the Word file name that held what I called a "journal" (but was really just a diary) that originated in 2021, just before my wife Shannon Beavers Woodruff was diagnosed with Lewy Body Dementia.

This is not a book about that cruel disease. There are folks who know far more about the medical aspects of it than I do, and there is a lot of information available on the internet for those who want it. This book is not about the disease so much as its progression and impact.

At the time of her diagnosis, we knew only that it was a terminal disease, a Parkinson's Disease variant, combining movement disorder and gradual physical failure with dementia.

She had her first visible symptoms - occasional confusion, lapses of memory, and frustration in 2019, and two years later she sought diagnosis/treatment.

It was clear at the time that the symptoms would worsen, though we had no estimated timeline for her expected decline. This illness is typified by wild swings in condition, from "pretty good" to "oh, shit!" daily, weekly, or even monthly, and known to last five to ten years… though those estimates are confused by the question of exactly when the disease began. That might be difficult to determine in the heat of the battle. Later, it may be somewhat easier with the benefits of hindsight.

My experience, and that of many caretakers to whom I have spoken, was "about three years, five at the most, from obvious symptoms and diagnosis to death." Many patients, experience an "episode" somewhat earlier, sometimes more than five years before diagnosis. But, from the moment the patient or loved ones realize that help is needed, a period of about three to five years is typical. I have come to regard it as "the disease of a thousand days." One thousand days from seeking help to grave.

So, my journal was a way of monitoring and recording Shannon's fight with this monstrous illness. I now know that there were times when the journal was my best friend. To it, I could confess or complain. I could express my aches and heartaches. I could disclose. In the first days, I could even hope, and no one would know unless I told them.

The keeping of the journal was prompted by my need for structure in a world that had none. I wanted a record of what Shannon was experiencing. Many years of management in the world's most litigious business – real estate – have taught me the value of "contemporaneous notes." I thought there could come a time when, for reasons unknown at the time, I might need to verify details I could no longer remember. A fatal disease might raise issues from many fronts, and a written record could come in handy. As it turned out, an unanticipated benefit of the journal was that it made it much easier to notify Shannon's family of her condition. I could simply copy an entry and paste it into an email. In this way, I did not have to rewrite the information to keep the family updated.

In writing this book and re-living each entry, the journal has become my enemy. It dredged up a recent and astonishingly painful three years. One thousand days in hell and heartache. Yet, it was also one thousand days of doing something very important.

MOST of this book is plucked directly from the journal, and most of THAT is simple diary entries, offered to the reader in unpolished form. Those entries suffer from the clipped descriptions, short entries, repetitions, and lack of context that are common to diaries. The entries also reveal my ignorance in many cases. I might have jumped to conclusions, made invlid assumptions, or simply been uninformed. Still, though they might be revealing of my stupidity, they are presented to you in whole cloth. Un-edited from the day they were written, though I was tempted often to "revise." But, revision would equal disrespect, robbing them of their immediacy and honesty. When those entries require expanded context, it is provided in "Digressions" that stop the progress in order to provide it. I have used real names in most cases. Shannon's childrens' and grandchildrens' names are aliases.

Those diary entries are sometimes just the day's thoughts and can be joyous, petty, angry, or even informative. In other cases, a single entry may attempt to synthesize two weeks or more into a few paragraphs. They may praise or criticize, and they are sometimes filled with anger and despair. In those cases, I have now put my regrets, grudges, and hopelessness behind me. So, if you read that I was "really pissed off" about something, well, I got over it. Probably. (See Chapter One, A Place for Mom.)

A cousin told me about a conversation with a loved one's physician. Treating a terminal illness, the physician said to her, "Be careful, this disease can rip a family apart." Yes, it can - and it did. The stress, financial burden, and hopelessness of a terminal illness can cause everyday folks like you and me to implode. Evolution did not equip us with some of the tools called for in the twenty-first century. If you are a caretaker or loved one of a dementia patient, prepare for a life-altering experience. Your patience will be tested, and you will either pass the test or perish inside. Your kindness will be stretched and either bloom or wither into despair and hatred. You will experience emotions that you cannot name. Hopelessness beyond your understanding. Immeasurable heartache. And, hopefully, at some time in the future, the most profound satisfaction you have ever known.

I do not envy your challenge. But I do understand it. Good luck to you.

Chapter 1
A Place for Mom

I wish I didn't know now what I didn't know then.
Bob Seger

March 2, 2024

Shannon awoke this morning inside a hallucination. Being "inside" a hallucination is different from "having" a hallucination. When Shannon had hallucinations, they were brief. "Did you see that bird fly into the bathroom?" "What are those kids doing camping out in the car?" With calming words from me, the hallucination would end. I could always "talk her down." Since the first of them in 2020, I had developed a method… a tone of voice… a calmness that calmed her, too. (Note that I was not calm – only sounded so.) This morning was different. Instead of seeing kids in the Toyota, she was interacting with them. She had become part of another world, and left mine behind.

She addressed me as "Daddy" and asked me to tell Mamma that the cornbread was done. She wanted to go to the neighborhood gates to make sure that her deceased sister Patti could get into the neighborhood. She was certain that we were planning to host a wedding for a friend who lives in Natchez, Mississippi. "Where is everyone going to sleep? We shouldn't be in the same bed together… what will the guests think when they find us in the same bed?" It did not matter what I said or how calmly I said it. She was determined, and when I tried to calm her, she accused me of gaslighting her and trying to make her think she was crazy.

"No, honey, you are NOT crazy. You are just sick. Can I get you to go back to bed?"

"I am NOT going back to bed. Not until you get those birds to quit rattling the windows."

"Ok, I'll scare them away."

"Why won't you tell me the truth about anything? Where is Patti? Where is Mamma?"

This went on all day, and she was still in the hallucination and still berating me hours after sundown. Since it was Saturday, no one in the medical community was answering their phone. We could typically communicate with Dr. Hillary Williams, her wonderful neurologist, through the hospital's patient portal, but that would not happen on a Saturday. There was no help coming, no cavalry on the horizon… we were in this until Monday morning at the soonest.

There have been a few times in my life that I have faced a frightening situation completely alone. Times when I realized that only my own wits and ability could keep me alive. Flying my Cessna through a moonless night with lightning on the horizon, my first time on the starting grid of a motorcycle race… at these times, there was an indescribable feeling in my chest. Not exactly fear, but not far from it. This was one of those times.

I did not sleep that Saturday night. Shannon resisted going to bed until later than usual and then absolutely crashed at about 9PM. We lay down together, I read her a few pages of a Paul McCartney biography, and when I glanced at her she was asleep – her first respite of the day. I watched TV until about 4AM, then tried but failed to nap.

March 3, 2024

Sunday was better than Saturday, though the hallucination continued. It seemed that she was calmer and more resigned. Getting her dressed and into the car took an hour of encouragement. We made the usual Sonic run. She ordered a small cheeseburger, which she did not finish, and a chocolate shake, which she did. We drove to a spot on the lake that she called "the dock of the bay." We watched a few boaters and ducks, trying to talk gently with one another. I had long ago given up on those intimate talks we once had… now, I just hoped that she would not ask, "Why me? Why did I get this? What did I do to deserve this?"

Sunday night brought the most frightening event, thus far, of her illness. The day itself was uneventful, though the hallucination continued. She was still convinced that we were hosting a wedding and that the guests would be horrified if they found us in the same bed. On Sunday night, after a dinner of salmon and asparagus which I ate and she nibbled, we were passing one another in the hallway. I watched as she leaned against the rock wall of the fireplace and heard her say, "Dave… come…"

I took two steps to reach her as she collapsed. She had fainted, and I wrapped my arms around her below her armpits to hold her upright. As she went completely limp, her arms stretched toward the ceiling, leaving me with no purchase, no grip on her. She fell through my arms to the floor, landing on her butt before falling onto her back, her eyes rolling backward within their sockets. She was flat on her back, eyes open but only the whites visible, unconscious and breathing shallowly. For an unclear period of time… less than a minute, I stood almost motionless, in a hopeless confusion. Do I call 911? Do I try to move her? Is she dying? With all these questions swirling in my mind, I soaked a towel in the coldest water in the house, right out of the fridge. I wanted her to awaken, I wanted a normal response to something, so I squeezed a cup or so of that frigid water from the towel onto her face. But she did not react and remained motionless. After what seemed like minutes, but was probably less than one, and only a moment before I called 911, her eyes began to flutter, then her pupils were again visible.

"Wha…what happened" she managed to squeak.

"You blacked out. How do you feel? Jeez… are you OK… I am going to call 911," I managed to say.

But Shannon said, "No, please… I'm ok now." Ten minutes later, we were sitting side by side on the couch and counting our blessings, though few they seemed. I was thrilled that her life did not end that way. We were… I was… settling for less and less as her disease progressed.

Her disease was diagnosed as Lewy Body Dementia, or LBD. As a Parkinson's Disease variant, to the tremors and other physical manifestations that accompany that horrible disease, LBD adds terminal mental and physical decline. It is a vicious and cruel disease; among the worst I can name. Like other dementias, it begins slowly, with symptoms possibly remaining hidden for years. Sleep disorders are common, but the patient's friends may not see any changes in the patient's personality until much closer to the final stages.

Ultimately, as the Lewy Bodies accumulate in the brain, dementia gathers strength. Names, dates, directions, and particularly math become more difficult and eventually impossible. In advanced cases, hallucinations often render the patient helpless. That is where we were – the advanced stages.

The disease is characterized by frequent ups and downs. Hourly. Daily. Even month to month, the patient's mood, hallucinations, and misunderstandings vary. In this way, LBD differs from Alzheimer's Disease, which is more of a "steady state" without the physical body failings of LBD. No two LBD patients travel the exact same path, but all go in the same direction, and all end the same way.

There is, frustratingly, no objective way to diagnose LBD. The Lewy Bodies themselves can be found in the brain only when autopsied. The diagnosis is, therefore, purely subjective, allowing only a sliver of hope to patients and loved ones– maybe the doctor is wrong. There is no blood test, no imaging, and no objective measure by which to say for sure that the patient is afflicted with LBD.

March 5, 2024

Monday morning, and I am on the phone before Shannon awakens. After a few calls… to the neurologist, the clinic, her psychiatrist, and the insurance company. I determined that the Emergency Room at Baptist Health Center was the place to go. IF she awakened in the same state of mind in which she went to sleep. Which, of course, she did. The hallucination continued. The same wedding. The same fear of getting caught in bed together. The same concerns about where the guests would sleep and whether the house was clean, and, and, and…

I was relieved when Shannon asked if I thought she should go to the hospital.

"Yes, we can go to the Emergency Room this afternoon. Are you OK with that?"

"I think we should go. I'll pack."

Of course, I knew that she would need little packing, but I said nothing. She filled a suitcase and a huge bag with enough supplies and clothes for a week in Hawaii. We left for the ER at about 1PM and arrived there an hour later. The staff was cordial and professional. There were wristbands, blood draws, endless questionnaires, and a lot of "get ready for…" and then "well, there's been a delay." At about 7PM, after sitting in the ER for five hours, the nurses and orderlies loaded her, dressed only in a hospital gown, into a van and departed for the Geriatric Behavioral Health Care Unit of Baptist Health Center (BHC) in Little Rock, Arkansas. As I watched the van drive into the darkness, I realized that Shannon would not be coming home. She was gone, and I was alone.

March 18, 2024

The Behavioral Unit of Baptist Hospital was an hour's drive from our home. I traveled there every day for two weeks for the visiting hour at 2PM. Her physical condition was frightening and worsening. She wanted to leave, to go home. She cried and begged and demanded to return to our home in Karnack or Houston or Dallas… wherever her current hallucination told her we were living that day. I always said "no" in the gentlest way possible. It was heartbreaking. Eventually, she said, "You promised to take care of me!"

"That's what I am doing."

"No, you're not. I am up here all alone, the nurses hate me. Last night, they killed a dog right there in that corner."

"Darling, all I can do is make sure that you are being cared for by the best nurses and doctors I can find. I just cannot care for you now. I can't keep you safe."

March 25, 2024

On the second Saturday after her admission, I visited and found her daughter, Bev, sitting in the community room awaiting Shannon. I did not expect her and had no previous notice of her visit.

She and I were quarreling, and I was particularly upset with her husband. It probably says enough that she was in town without my knowledge and that she and her husband were shopping for a nursing home. Brad, her son, was busy in Arizona with his contribution, an Excel Spreadsheet of different nursing homes, complete with ratings, addresses, and whether or not they locked down "wanderers" (those patients with a propensity to leave their rooms and roam, zombie-like, through the facility.) I am not sure what he was notating, but it was surely limited to facts that he could gather through a Google search.

I was ambivalent about this, as well as Bev's visit. I was grateful for any help, whether obtained under duress or even if it was help of no consequence. Still, I was surprised to find that their criteria for selecting a temporary home for their mother did not include an Excel spreadsheet column for "How far is it from David?" It was clear that neither she nor her brother were concerned about whether or not I could easily visit their mother. It must be noted at this time that none of us knew (or even guessed) that her time was so limited. We were thinking, all of us, about a home for years. It turned out to be weeks. We got weeks.

A month or two earlier, we had submitted an application to Brandon Autrey, the Business Office Manager at Belvedere Nursing Home. (Attempting to build rapport with Mr. Autrey, I asked if he was related to the famous cowboy singer, Gene Autrey. Surprisingly, he said, "Yes, he was my third cousin or uncle or something like that.") Belvedere is a magnificent, nearly new facility only ten miles from my home. It was perfect, and Shannon was approved for early (pre-Medicaid approval) entry, but no rooms were available.

April 1, 2024

I am now going to take the reader through the frustrating and depressing search for a comfortable place for Shannon to live out her last months or even years. Warning: if I communicate this section properly, the reader will feel my frustration and anger at the incompetence, rudeness, and dismissiveness of certain people with whom I met, as well as the bizarre nature of the "information" that I received from them. Of particular significance were:

Quapaw Nursing Home, Hot Springs, Connie

The Blossoms Nursing Home at Hot Springs, Tonya

The Blossoms Nursing Homes General Management, Little Rock, Joanna.

Anna Freeman, the quietly competent shift supervisor at the Behavioral Unit phoned me. They had done all they could for Shannon, and it was time for her discharge. What was I doing to find a place for her? I did not know how to answer because it was surprisingly difficult to find "a place for Mom."

As background, I should relate a few items of context. Upon Shannon's diagnosis, I engaged attorneys who specialize in elder care. They drew a "living will" for Shannon to control her health destiny and a Power of Attorney for me to sign in Shannon's place when she became unable to understand for herself. They also gave us a "primer" on the legal requirements we should understand.

The most important of these is related to **Medicaid.** Medicaid is easy to understand, but very difficult to obtain. Medicaid would, at that time, cover the expense of nursing home long-term care, subject to the following rules.

1. The patient can have no personal assets beyond $2000 in cash or checking/savings accounts. (This is rigorously checked, bank statements for both husband and wife are required to go back for several months… eight in Shannon's case. PayPal and Zelle usages and statements are examined. Insurance policies are examined. Any place imaginable, where one can park money is reviewed. Closed accounts must be proven to be closed. Zelle transfers must be explained. Tax certificates must be furnished. MARRIAGE LICENSE! They leave no stone unturned.
2. If the patient is married, the assets and income of the spouse **are not considered**. The patient can have one car (many married people title their vehicles in BOTH of their names… e.g., David Legan and Shannon Woodruff), and a car thus titled is "one car in the patient's name." If the married couple owns two cars titled in this way, they must sell one of those cars in order to qualify for Medicaid. Having seen the drama imposed on a couple we knew with a deceased spouse, Shannon and I titled the cars and motorcycles in the name of David Legan OR Shannon Woodruff. If either of us was dead or incapacitated, the other was able to do anything necessary to sell the vehicles, with no artificial limitations imposed by the title(s). So, we would be allowed to keep the two cars.
3. The patient must be otherwise eligible… age 65 or more, a participant in Medicare, the simple stuff.

Cars and other assets, and my income were not problems… if everyone understood the rules as I did.

They did not. In fact, I was bewildered at the amount of misinformation that I was provided by folks who, I had assumed, dealt with this subject on a daily basis. My surprise would turn to despair before the end.

My first stop was at Quapaw, the corporate sister facility of Belvedere. I met there with a lovely woman who repeatedly said, "If she meets our criteria." I should have been alarmed by her repetition of this phrase… it was almost as if she was preparing me for a disappointing outcome. Belvedere and Quapaw were facilities that meet most people's definition of a "great place for Mom." Bright colors, impeccable housekeeping, no strange odors. (A friend who had spent years in the nursing home business told me, "Pick the one with the least smell of urine…") So, I held out great hope for Quapaw, until Connie informed me that they "Could not meet Shannon's needs."

"Why is that?" I asked.

"We just cannot meet her needs."

"Is it a problem with her condition?" I asked. "Is it Medicaid?"

"We simply cannot meet her needs."

"Yes, you said that. I just want to know why. I'm not gonna argue with you, but I need to know. Now. Why."

No change in the response or tone.

I then told Connie, the Office Manager, that I needed Shannon's life insurance policy returned to me. (I had been, unfortunately, in a hurry on application day, and I had not made my own copy. My fault.) She said that she did not have it, that she had never had it, and dismissed me. It was not the last time that I would be dismissed.

I will admit to becoming angry at this time, but I departed, in deepening confusion, without the insurance policy. About five minutes into the drive home, I received a call from a gentleman who worked in the office. He said, “Mr. Legan, we made a digital copy of your entire application, and I can give you a copy of your insurance policy.”

“Great,” I replied and returned to Quapaw. Connie was gone for the day.

A few days later, I realized that I needed the ORIGINAL cover page of the insurance policy, and all I had was a copy. I called and reached Connie. Almost angrily, she said, “I already told you that I do not have it and never did!”

I said, “Your colleague gave me a copy of it, from your files, so we both know you had it. I’m not trying to make things hard on you, but I actually NEED it. It is a Medicaid thing. I NEED the original.”

“Well, that’s your business… I cannot help you.”

I was exasperated, and so I said, in the softest voice I could summon, “Connie, I am trying to find a place for my wife to die. Why are you being so rude and dismissive to me? Have I offended you in some way?”

There was an audible sigh from her end of the phone, and I was now talking to an entirely different Connie. “Oh, Mr. Legan. I’m frazzled and did not mean to be rude.”

“Well, you were actually quite rude.” I was going to let her off the hook, but not quite that easily.

“I know, and I apologize. I have looked everywhere for your documents, and the copies we furnished you are the best we can do.”

She was, or at least sounded, sincere. I thanked her and wrote to the insurer for a copy of the policy. It could not be sent by overnight delivery, even if I paid the fifteen bucks. Postal service only. The heavens and earth were conspiring to delay this process and make it as difficult as possible. The application was already hundreds of pages long and would get MUCH longer.

Ms. Freeman, one of the most helpful of the professionals with whom I dealt, recommended that I talk with Joanna, an executive with The Blossoms, a corporation that operates several Arkansas facilities.

I had already spoken with Tonya, a middle-aged woman with the rugged skin of a long-term smoker, the Business Office Manager at The Blossoms at Hot Springs. The outcome there was remarkably similar to that of Quapaw. Tonya had been very positive at our initial interview, sitting behind her desk with her cigarette within reach, awaiting the "smoke break" which was allowed to residents and employees alike.

But when I stopped in to see how things were progressing, she refused to see me! Flummoxed, I was hanging around in the waiting room when a nurse wearing a stiffly starched uniform arrived.

She said, "We cannot meet her needs."

Oh, no. Not this again!

"Why is that?" I asked.

"We simply cannot meet her needs."

"Is it her condition, qualifying for Medicaid? What?"

After a couple more rounds of this, I asked, "Are you married?"

"I don't think that's relevant," she replied.

"And you are correct. It's not relevant. But IF you were married, and IF your husband was dying, you would not be afraid of insulting a tight-ass nurse like yourself."

Back to the car.

On the recommendation of Ms. Freeman, I phoned Joanna, of the Blossoms corporate management. Having already lost my taste for the company, thanks to Tonya and Nurse Starch, I was leery. It was about to get worse. Upon hearing a few details, Joanna informed me that Shannon did not qualify for Medicaid! What?!? Of course she does! I've got a lawyer, I've spoken to a half dozen lawyers. I know these rules!

"No, sir. You receive a monthly retirement payment of $4000, which disqualifies her."

"NO IT DOES NOT!" I was almost shouting. "The patient is qualified based on the **patient's** income and assets." I stammered, stung by her ignorance on this vital topic.

"In Arkansas, that's not how we do it. What's yours is hers and vice versa."

This statement is SO incorrect that I was speechless, feeling as if I had been transported to an alternate universe. We were not talking about real estate law here… I know about community property and dower rights – Jeez, I'm a Realtor. This was FEDERAL POLICY! She might as well have said, "Actually, you are in Italy, not the United States. Has no one informed you?" She was incredibly dismissive, her tone conveying that I must be the most stupid human on earth.

I was nearing panic. How could I be SO wrong about this? I consulted with another attorney. He confirmed that I was correct, and that for a fee of $4,800, he could "make them see the light." Though I was right, it looked like I might be forced to divorce Shannon if she was to get the help she required. Once he took his $4,800 and showed the light to Joanna, she could simply say, "We cannot meet her needs," I surmised.

It was then I decided that regardless of the consequences, these people were wrong, and I knew how to prove it. My logic went like this: I am not a rich man. There were no hidden gems or bonds. I was a common guy facing a very common problem. Shannon was a Medicare and Social Security recipient. She had no assets to speak of and was facing a terminal and disabling disease for which I was incapable of serving as a caretaker.

Medicaid was created for precisely this situation, and there was no possibility that our federal government would create a policy that encouraged husbands to divorce their ailing wives. FHA, the Veterans Administration, SNAP, on and on… all exhibitions of our government's commitment to strengthening families. Why? The cynic would say, "That's the best way to keep income taxes high," while the idealist would say, "That's the best way to promote a strong society." Both would be correct.

The final step in my logic was this: Private care, paid for by the patient, costs about $9,000 monthly. Even if I devoted ALL of our income, my four thousand plus about two thousand eight hundred dollars of Social Security between the two of us, even if we spent 100% of our available funds on a nursing home, it would still not be enough. That simply could not be the government's policy. Period.

But it would not matter.

It would not matter because, just as I was losing all hope, a man named Claude Mahend, an executive with the Blossoms Corporation, would return a panic-stricken message that I left at his office. Their corporate website listed two phone numbers at that time. The general business number did not answer. Ever. Thirty tries, no answer. The other number specified that it was for "complaints only." There, I left a rambling and desperate message. I was a helpless and disheartened man, pleading for a return call from someone… anyone with the ability to hear MY side and help. Mr. Mahend made it clear, immediately, that he would help. "I am in Memphis on business" he said. "But one of my associates relayed your message to me and told me, "Claude, you gotta hear this."

When I mentioned Ms. Craig, he paid her the highest of compliments. He said that she is "mom" to all of Blossoms and a fine Vice President or whatever. I told him that she was incredibly wrong about the income/assets thing. He said, "Go check the Health and Human Resources Regulations, and call me back with language that proves your assertions." BINGO. Now, we are getting somewhere. I called him back in less than five minutes and read him this: "When only one spouse is an applicant, only the applicant spouse's income is counted. This means the income of the non-applicant spouse is not used in determining income eligibility of their spouse…"

I did not need to convince Mr. Mahend. He did not see our discussion as an argument. He was not at all interested in being right. He wanted to help. "We cannot meet her needs" is not in his vocabulary. He said, "If you promise to deliver her bank statements for the last six months, I will admit her this week."

April 4, 2024

After three days at home in Hot Springs Village, I drove Shannon to The Blossoms of Midtown (Little Rock), where the staff greeted her with appropriate enthusiasm.

A critical step in Shannon's care was complete. It was done. Over the next couple of weeks, I would add a refrigerator and comfortable chairs to her room, as well as a plastic chair in which to sit while showering in her private bath. Bev came to our home and selected framed photos from our walls to make the room seem homier. Her room was just across the corridor from the nurses' station. The food was edible, though not fancy. The facility was odor-free and well-kept. It was a great place for mom.

Even Bev approved.

Chapter 2
Before the Storm

The trouble is, you think you have time
Jack Kornfield

Each of us came a long way to reach this place in our lives. She was married for thirty-five years and raised two grown children. Me, married 30 years, with three adult children. All five were college-educated and independent.

She and I met in 1966 at Woodlawn High School in Shreveport, Louisiana. But we only really met through Facebook in 2011, both of us 61 at the time.

I have ridden motorcycles since 1963. In high school I rode a sportbike that had a tendency to break down frequently due to teenager abuse. During our junior year, I bought (with earnings from McDonald's) a much larger bike and it was even worse, sitting silently in the garage more days than not. So, with an unreliable motorcycle and factoring in rain and cold, I rode the school bus often, and Shannon rode it, too. (So did one of the finest football players in the history of the game, Terry Bradshaw, who lived only three blocks from my home.)

I did not know Shannon, but I knew of her. Every student in school did. She was one of those girls that a guy like me looks at and thinks, "No way, she's out of my league." So, we had not known one another as high schoolers. Though we would attend the same school and ride the same bus for three years, we never had a conversation. Shannon would later say that she remembered me as the kid who was constantly arguing with someone about something. (I was on the debate team, partnering with Gary Hayes, about whom you will learn more in this book.)

Shannon's son, Brad, is a father of two, a son and a daughter, both not quite teens at that time. Both are very bright. Shannon was a grandparent! Fifteen years ago, and she was already something I am not, even now. Her son Brad and his family live in Arizona, where Brad, a PhD, was (and remains) a professor at a state university. His wife is a lovely, intelligent, and politically active woman – an attentive mother to their children- and a professional in her own right.

Shannon's daughter, Bev, obtained a master's degree in Texas. When we left Shreveport in 2013, she was working on her PhD at Stanford and living in San Francisco. She lived in the cool part of town, had a cool apartment, and a cool job as an intern with Kaiser Permanente. Pretty cool, huh?

Shannon was very proud of her children. She and her husband, Danny, raised two well-educated and focused adults during a time of crazy fluctuations in the oil business in which Danny worked. They had lived in:

Natchez, Mississippi;

Dallas, Texas;

Tulsa, Oklahoma;

Shreveport, Louisiana;

Houston, Texas;

Some of them more than once. They relocated frequently because oil prices ranged from ten dollars to one hundred dollars a barrel, and Danny was subject to the whims of that industry. Along the way, Shannon discovered that she had a talent for the fashion retail business. She worked for Nordstrom's Department Stores for two decades in Houston, Dallas, and later, Scottsdale, Arizona.

She was accustomed to relocating and traveling. In fact, she was the best travel companion I have ever known. She was a TRAVEL MONSTER, feeling at home only when she was not. We traveled in the motorhome for four years, and Shannon would still be in it if she had her way.

I had three children. My daughter Macy, 29 at the time, was a speech therapist, working on her master's degree in Mobile, Alabama. A son, Hank, was two years her junior, and a property manager in Austin. Another son, David, who was two years younger, lived in Little Rock, Arkansas, and worked for the United States Department of Agriculture when he wasn't skydiving. We would, at one time or another, stop to see all of our children at their homes.

We had no mission except to drive from one adventure to the next, from one luscious destination to the next. That October evening, we were headed for Phoenix. We had driven all day and into the night just to get across Texas.

Somewhere in New Mexico, as I drove that lumbering motorhome (towing a cute red Jeep with a green Kawasaki Ninja motorcycle on its bumper) through the darkness, I turned to her and said, "I can't believe we are getting to do this." Neither of us could believe it. As a real estate broker, I had worked for twenty-five years with a total of thirty days of vacation time. Both of us now felt somehow guilty and undeserving of this enormous gift.

Where were we going? First to Phoenix and the surrounding mountains, then to the Pacific Coast Highway. After that? We did not know. We would turn right or left at the ocean and see what lay over the next hill.

Shannon's daughter, Bev, finished her PhD at Stanford and was settled in San Francisco. So, we turned right and spent three glorious months on the coast, just south of her. Olema, then Half Moon Bay, the SLO coast - San Luis Obispo area- just south of Bev. Alice's Restaurant was just over the hills to the east. The roads were motorcycle-ready, and Shannon had the Jeep to commute to Bev's home, where she stayed a month. We spent the deep winter and early spring there, including our second Christmas. New Year's Eve was danced away to a grade B Tom Petty "tribute" band.

Most days, when Shannon was in San Franciso, I rode my little Ninja motorcycle about a hundred miles, north and south on Pacific Coast Highway, the uncontested winner of the "most beautiful ride in this country award." Southbound, the Pacific Ocean with its seals and otters is on the right, and rocky cliffs tower above on the left. It is breathtaking, as it had been the first time I had ridden it, in 1972. Like the Grand Canyon, it is a place I return to every few years to renew my soul… well, at least my attitude.

After wearing out the Pacific Coast Highway and the San Luis Obispo coastline, we drove south. Bev rode with us, stopping to disembark and join friends in Los Angeles. We were traveling to Chula Vista, about two miles from Mexico. Beautiful place. Marina, excellent restaurants with live music, a pool, and an enormous hot tub on the campground. This is called glamping, and we took to it quickly. We attended a concert in the intimate back room of McCabe's Guitar

Store in Santa Monica, where we saw one of my songwriting heroes, Jack Tempchin (who wrote Peaceful Easy Feeling for the Eagles), accompanied by Chris Hillman (founder of the rock group The Byrds) sitting within whispering distance of them. We also attended two Neil Young concerts, saw James Taylor at the Hollywood Bowl, and the Eagles in San Jose, California. Now, that is about as cool as it gets… The Eagles in San Jose! I needed new sunglasses.

Two months there, and we headed north again, still on the PCH, then Interstate Highway 5. Along that ride, somewhere in the high desert with traffic bumper to bumper at 90mph, our passenger window blew out! It was a replacement unit, made of plexiglass, and it simply exited the motorhome, making a frightening sound as it flew away. I stopped on the shoulder and walked backward at least a quarter mile to find it. I trudged back in the desert sun and found a roll of tape in the toolbox. It required so much tape to hold the window in place that we looked much like Grapes of Wrath movie extras – on our way to the promised land.

We spent a week in Mendicino County – the reputed capital of marijuana (of course, I know NOTHING about that) in the United States - and from there continued north. A couple of weeks in Oregon included a few days at the incredible Crater Lake. This collapsed volcano is about six thousand years old, dated by the moccasins of Indigenous Americans found in its rubble. There are no creeks or rivers feeding Crater Lake, its crystal blue water is 100% snowmelt. On the way inland, near the park, we noticed VERY tall poles sticking from the ground on both sides of the road. We were puzzled but thought little of it. That night, we had dinner in the lodge. A pamphlet promoting the park was on our table, and I read that this area averaged four hundred fifty inches of snow per year. What!?! That is forty feet of snow. It was June, and there was still snow in the shadows. Then, we realized the purpose of the roadside poles. They marked the under-snow location of the roads!

It was glorious to discover these new places, with Shannon, at 64 years of age.

After a few more days on the road, we arrived in Seattle. It was June, warm and sunny, and many young people were downtown, showing off their untanned winter skin. The Pike Place fish market and the Space Needle are everything you have heard, but only worth a short visit to seasoned travelers like us. Seasoned travelers like us preferred our campfires!

Digression

At a campground in the mountains east of Los Angeles, we were approached by a camp manager who sold us a membership in Thousand Trails Campground Club. He explained that we could join for $150 per month and stay rent-free in their affiliated campgrounds located all over the U.S. There were many of those campgrounds, most located within 200 miles of a coastline. We found that we could cut our lot rental costs from about thirty dollars a night to a much smaller monthly fee. The only limitation was that our stay in any campground was limited to three weeks. Then, we would have to go somewhere else for a week before returning. In most states, certainly every state with a coastline, we could stay essentially forever, alternating between nearby Thousand Oaks campgrounds every three weeks. The three-week policy is a good one, intended to prevent a <u>motorhome</u> park from becoming a <u>mobile home</u> park, as many do.

My wrist had begun to hurt most of the time and tingle all of the time, and we stayed in the Seattle area long enough for me to undergo carpal tunnel surgery.

When told about our adventures, many of our friends and acquaintances remark, "Oh, we have ALWAYS wanted to do that!" If they only knew. There are many reasons NOT to go for a three-year vacation in a motorhome. Certainly, medical need is one of them. If I needed wrist surgery at home, I would call my PCP, and he would refer me to a specialist. I would see the specialist the next week and have surgery the next. It does not work like that when you are two thousand miles from home. I needed to first see a PCP, then she would refer me to an unknown specialist, and there would be test after test before surgery… about a two-month wait.

From the campground, I would ride the little Ninja into the city, park in the underground facility beneath one of the many buildings of Virginia-Mason Medical Center, and take a few steps to the check-in desk. They were always ready for me and sent me to the elevator. And when the elevator door opened for me to exit, there was ALWAYS an orderly or nurse waiting for me.

"Mr. Legan?"

"Yes, that's me."

"Please follow me, Sir."

And this person would lead me to an exam room where I would wait a maximum of two minutes before being seen by a nurse or physician. It was The. Finest. Service. I have ever experienced, period. Service like this engenders trust, and I had no problem entrusting my wrist to the surgeons there.

They told me that the anesthesia would be a "local," and, realizing that I would be awake to watch, I asked if they would allow me to cut the tendon myself! "NO," they said, and fearing my impulsiveness, they put me under. I awoke with a dead right arm. Shannon drove us back to the campground. I had delayed at least six months after realizing that something was wrong with my wrist, and for that delay, I paid. I permanently lost the fine motor movement of my right hand. I can hold handlebars. I can hold a golf club. But I cannot hold a guitar pick. That's a price that I continue to pay.

East of Seattle are two exquisite towns named Issaquah and Snoqualmie. With the Thousand Oaks membership, and three qualifying campgrounds in the Seattle area (one in the Snoqualimie area), we were there for the entire summer of 2014. We rode ferries through Saget Bay and Peugeot Sound, watched the Doobie Brothers outdoors in a city park, and twice ate dinner at a theatre/restaurant while watching guitarist Alvin Lee and the cast of Playing for Change (go Grandpa Jones!) as we ate steak and drank cocktails, comfortably sitting in Michelin class seats.

We visited Mount Baker and Mount Ranier, both gorgeous snow-covered conical mountains rising from surprisingly flat surroundings. Both were formed by the "hot spot" of volcanic activity that moved northward with a tectonic plate over millions of years.

We aimed the motorhome southeastward in August 2014. Crossing the country took a month or so, and we stopped to visit several friends and national parks along the way. The Arches. Pikes Peak. Kent (rip) and Mary Phelps in Colorado, Reid Miller in Wisconsin, Sue Gauthier in Kentucky, and my son David at a skydiving park in Tennessee. We also stopped for the Sturgis Motorcycle Rally in South Dakota, the Rock and Roll Hall of Fame Museum in Cleveland, the Corvette Museum in Bowling Green and Beale Street in Memphis. We considered continuing east from Chicago to Niagara Falls and then Maine but did not (and I still regret it.) I had violated Legan's Law Number Three – be very careful about passing over an opportunity that may never come again.

Back in Shreveport, we watched LSU football games at the magnificent home of Gary and Patricia Hayes, my friends since 1966. Then, as winter set in, we slipped out again with the GPS guiding us to Florida. Snowbirds! We arrived there just in time for "fresh-squeezed orange juice season" and left in March after the Daytona 200 Motorcycle race.

Along the journey, I bought and sold two or three really expensive Martin guitars and motorcycles, and to Shannon's credit, she never complained. "You REALLY love that thing, don't you," she said as I massaged a forty-year-old Martin D-76 rosewood guitar in Kissimmee, Florida.

While in Florida, we accepted a long-standing invitation to visit Jeff Rogers and his wife Izzy on their fifty-two-foot yacht, the Izzy R, in the Virgin Islands. What a life they lived! They were "island hoppers," motoring gently from one to the next, Jeff and I ensuring we did not pass a single saloon. We spent a week enjoying the most beautiful ocean I had ever seen, and the relentless hospitality of Jeff and Izzy. They spent ten years in the Caribbean, and we were lucky to get them home to Orange County, California, in 2019.

During the journey, there was not a single discouraging word from Shannon, despite tirades of my profanity when something went wrong with the house on wheels. As I have written, she was a travel monster. Shannon did not exhibit, during this time, any symptoms of her disease, though it was almost certainly in its earliest stages. She DID have a tendency toward very active dreams, which I now realize were signs of coming dementia. Our bodies are supposed to become paralyzed during REM sleep. Acting out, thrashing, shouting, and rolling about are not common REM actions. But, not knowing otherwise, we would laugh when I repeated the things she said in her dreams.

One night, as she was sleeping and I was reading beside her, she began to fight unknown demons in her dream. She literally shouted out, "Get off of my floor, you bitch. You are going down!" I shook her awake, repeated the story, and we both laughed. That, or something similar, happened scores of times over the next six years. And it was always funny… until it wasn't.

By the summer of 2016, we were somewhat tired of stashing and deploying electrical lines, water hoses, and sewer conduits. Drive to a new destination, find a good spot, park just so to get a good TV reception, extend the hoses and lines, wash, rinse, repeat. I wanted a garage and something other than a little Ninja and a Jeep to fill it. After thinking it through, we decided to buy a home in a place where other people went on vacation. We looked at homes in Florida and considered some in Dallas. We settled on Hot Springs Village, Arkansas, about halfway between Little Rock and Hot Springs. With eight lakes, nine golf courses, walking trails… 13,000 people on 25,000 acres, gates at the east and west ends were connected by a sixteen-mile-long road that bisected the largest gated community in the nation.

We had no furniture; everything had either been sold or damaged by flooding while in storage. So, we looked for a former VRBO home and found one… furnished all the way down to the silverware, with an enormous deck overlooking hundreds of forested acres. Moving in was a matter of introducing our two Maine Coon cats, Buddy and Cricket, to their new home, and buying new linens.

Digression

As a property manager in 2011 I met a family who was moving to Guam because of an Air Force re-assignment. They had several cars and motorcycles, a flock of children, and a herd of pets… all of which (except the kids) they were selling or giving away. I am a cat lover and had lost a long-time companion, 17-year-old Lissie, a few months prior. These folks introduced me to Maine Coons Murphy (orange male) and Leila (white female.) They were fully grown young adults, brother and sister, totally socialized from their adventures in this circus of a household, and I took them home that night. I re-named them Buddy and Cricket, in honor of Buddy Holly and the Crickets, and they settled in quickly. They rode with us in the motorhome, which

Shannon had named "Homer" in honor of her father, Homer Beavers. They adjusted well. During our first trip (a shakedown cruise), from Shreveport to Charlie and Kathy Grau's home in Virginia Beach, Cricket escaped at a state park in Georgia, and did not return to Homer. We waited a couple of days, walking the park and calling "Crick-et, Crick-et," but she did not show up. We left the park after giving the camp manager our contact info and her photo. Two months later, as we were enjoying Carefree, (yes, really) Arizona, he called. "I have your cat," he said. She was cold and thin from scrounging for herself in the Georgia pines for 65 days.

"Okay," I said. "Give me your address, and I'll send you fifty bucks for her food while I figure out what to do."

I located a woman in Jacksonville, Florida, who specialized in this sort of task. She drove to the park, retrieved Cricket, and had a veterinarian administer shots. Then, she bought a proper cage for an airliner and shipped her to Phoenix. Shannon and I drove to the freight office at Phoenix airport, where we found Cricket squalling like a demon inside her shipping crate. Buddy actually seemed angry with her. Raising hell, pacing back and forth, hissing at her. Of course, she hissed back, but by morning, all was forgiven. Until she did it again at Half Moon Bay, California.

We were there for a month, and I again printed flyers and walked the campground calling out to her, fruitlessly, for over a week. A young couple was tent camping in the spot next to us, and the gentleman said, "I think your cat comes back at night and checks out your motorhome. She hangs out a while, then leaves."

Aha, I thought, raccoon trap! The local ACE Hardware sold me one for thirty bucks, and I armed it with a can of cat food before setting the trap door that evening. The next morning, she was trapped and squalling like a banshee again. Again, Buddy chastised her before forgiving and resuming the grooming they did to one another. (Buddy grew into a 35-pound gentle giant, the heaviest cat ever weighed in Hot Springs Village, according to the vet. He died at 14 years of age while I was writing this book. Cricket soldiers along, refusing to even walk out on the deck, always stopping at the doorframe. She may have learned her lesson.

We were delighted newcomers in Hot Springs Village. In my last years before traveling, I was a decent and frequent golfer, carrying a six handicap for years. I played fairly well, won and lost many thousands of dollars, and had a LOT of fun. I was looking forward to reclaiming my lost skills, but never did. Sciatica drove me out of the game before Shannon became so very ill. From then on, there was no time for golf.

Shannon wanted to stay busy and found a part-time job at a gift shop near our home. It was there, in 2017, that she experienced the first episode (other than her crazy dreams) of the disease that would claim her life and rob us of our golden years. This beautiful, intelligent woman – this woman who had managed the entire "leather floor" of Nordstroms at the high-end North Park Galleria in Dallas, had melted down in front of a customer who needed change from a $19.65 purchase. This woman who had sold handbags for ten thousand dollars apiece could not count out thirty-five cents in change for a twenty-dollar bill. This was going to get indescribably worse.

That is what I will try to do in this book. Describe it.

Chapter 3
2021
Diagnosis

With your chrome heart shining in the sun, long may you run.
Neil Young

March 17, 2021

Shannon and I began to realize about two years ago, that her memory and mental function were declining. She had noticed it sooner and complained, but I did not see it. I thought she was exaggerating, possibly for selfish reasons. I was insensitive and dismissive. Don't get me wrong, here. I believe in being gentle with oneself, and I carry no residual guilt over this misjudgment. Nevertheless, I also believe in calling it what it was.

She began a series of visits to the doctors at the University of Arkansas Medical School (UAMS), Longevity Clinic, in February 2021. At that time, Shannon had experienced several incidents which concerned us. Two or three incidents of "negligent" car control, and at least one of semi-consciousness while in public.

In that instance, at Magellan Golf Course within The Village, she left the golf cart on foot and began to walk in circles beneath a large tree on a hillside. Walking uphill, she was slow and labored. But, when she turned downhill, she sped up to the point of almost falling, arms flailing in search of balance. She made two or three orbits as I chased after her, calling her name and demanding that she stop. She only stopped when I physically stopped her, and she "came to" as if exiting a trance.

There was test after test, each requiring a month or two of scheduling and then another visit to discuss the results. The round trip from our home to the hospital in Little Rock is 120 miles, and we made that trip over a dozen times in the first half of 2021.

March 19, 2021

Shannon has been getting more forgetful lately. She gets confused easily and seems to have accepted a "diagnosis" that she is in an early stage of dementia. She tells people about it. When her nephew Steve phoned, she told him immediately. At a furniture store, she took a call from UAMS and told her caller that she needed an MRI quickly because "I have been diagnosed with dementia," speaking in a voice loud enough for everyone in the building to hear. On vacation two days ago, she told my best friend, Charlie Grau. She later told me, "I was acting so stupid that I felt like I needed to explain." I've asked her not to tell people about it. She says that it is nothing to be ashamed of, and that is true. But it is also no one else's business, and I am, inexplicably, somewhat embarrassed for her. (I now realize that it was not embarrassment. It was denial.)

March 21, 2021

We returned today, two days early, from a short vacation. We went to see Charlie and his sailboat in Saint Petersburg, Florida, after stopping for the evening and a great dinner with Bev, her husband, and his son, Brian. Bev is concerned. I am too, but more than she. Until the vacation, I thought it might have been just BS. But, it's not. She did a LOT of weird things. Many involved waking from a dream, convinced that other people were nearby. She is often confused. She lost her phone and her wallet three times each –in the car- as we drove home. There's a pocket in her massive purse that is perfect for the wallet and phone. She agrees and promises to use it, then does not. She carries a lot of unnecessary stuff, such as an ice chest, bags of snacks, extra Blistex, sunglasses, blankets, and pillows, and she constantly munches. Tonight, after arriving home, she went to sleep immediately. Within 15 minutes, she was awake, shuffling through our home, asking me who else was in the house, and looking for Bev. She opened the front door and called out to Bev, presumably thinking that Bev was on our front lawn.

March 22, 2021

Shannon had a mixed weekend. On the $20^{th,}$ she tried to assemble her memories of the night before. She remembered me as her father... he shows up in many of these dreams. She was in a foul mood, but Bev phoned, and she perked up nicely. Saturday was then great. No problems. Until she asked me to reset the clock for Daylight Saving Time. She said that she had been trying for several minutes. I showed her the little wheel adjuster on the back. Move it, and the hands move. But that wasn't the problem. She had that figured out... she simply could not set the time to 2:25. She could not figure out the hand positions to indicate that time. Then she accused me of accusing her of "putting on." Maybe she had a right to feel that way because I thought it was impossible that she could not tell time! But we talked through it. I told her that I think she gives up too easily... even if she does have cognitive decline, I still expect her to refuse to give up. We had a good remainder of the day, but her stomach was upset by dinner at Acapulco Restaurant.

October 2, 2021

The day our lives changed.

Dr. Hillary Williams, or “Hill Will” as she is known, stood up behind her desk, took a deep breath, and began to step toward Shannon. As she stepped past the desk, she reached back and silently picked up a small package of tissues.

We met with Hill Will to discuss a tremor that had developed in Shannon’s right arm. Dr. Williams was in possession of all of Shannon’s previous tests and a lengthy psychological study. Those indicated a low level of dopamine and some reduction in mental acuity. After further questioning and testing Shannon, she was prepared to deliver a diagnosis. Now seated and facing Shannon knee to knee, she said, “You have Lewy Body Dementia. You have NOT changed. You are still Shannon Woodruff.” She delivered the diagnosis without providing information about what it meant to have LBD. That news was so awful that she could not bring herself to say the words. Those words were contained in pamphlets she provided.

LBD is progressive, aggressive, and terminal. Similar to Alzheimer’s in the dementia symptoms, and to Parkinsons in the movement disorder. (What I never read, what I was never told, is that the "movement disorder" is accompanied by physical decline, which ultimately takes the life of the patient.) It is a gruesome, brutal, and insidious disease, among the worst diseases imaginable. It has a typical course of five to ten years from the onset of symptoms, with an average of about six.

So, with typical progression, Shannon is three or four years away from the end.

October 6, 2021

I am not handling this as well as I must. I STILL become impatient with her. I STILL become annoyed at her declining capabilities and resistance to my efforts to "help." She has two hair care appointments this week and cannot keep them straight. This has driven her to tears of frustration amid feelings of impotence. Last night was terrible. All my fault. The details are not important, but the result is that I have made a renewed commitment to ease her burden. That's tough. She is growing more demanding. More "bitchy." More critical, more desirous of changing things around the house. Gotta move the Ficus trees into the house. Gotta blow off the leaves from the yard. Gotta, gotta, gotta. None of it matters in the grand scheme, but I must do ALL of it. Every time I hear her walking down the hall and calling "David," I know that there is some new project, errand, or task that she wants completed, and since she cannot do it, I will have to. I'll get better at handling this. She will get more difficult but less demanding. My burden will gradually shift from doing what she asks to helping with her personal care and hygiene. This will be a gradual shift and presage the end.

This diary is not about me, but I am being personally affected. Shannon's disease will end her life, and in doing so, it will end my active life. Yesterday, I went to the gym for an hour, leaving her at home. When I returned, she was hiding in her closet, frightened from hearing noises inside the house – possibly aural hallucinations – a first. She's not capable of taking care of herself already! So, the idea of taking a half day for a round of golf is out of the question. And the motorcycle, which has been the love of my life and provided my solitude and mental diversion/release/tranquility for almost sixty years, must sit quietly in the garage. I cannot risk riding it because an injury, even a small one, would leave me unable to tend to Shannon. By the time I can ride it again, I will probably be near or beyond 75 years of age. So, it is not an exaggeration to say that the end of Shannon's physical life coincides with the end of my active life. I'm not complaining. I'm simply remarking on the irony.

Digression

Shannon and I were driving to see her daughter Bev in Jackson, Mississippi. We were discussing one of the questions from the mental exam. "Count backwards from 100 by 7s." Jeez, what a question. It had perplexed Shannon to the point that she cried at the time and was still talking about it. Now, this is not to brag. Although I am actually very weak at math, but I am damned good at ARITHMETIC. As a motorcyclist I spent hundreds of hours playing arithmetic games, inspired by the road signs of distances to a coming town, in my head as I rode. "If Waco is 210 miles away, and I travel at 70mph, I can get there in three hours." I could add, subtract, calculate fractions and percentages in my head... more of a habit than a gift. And to be fair, Shannon and I had always been competitive when it came to many mind games... particularly rock and roll trivia, at which she was amazingly adept.

So, when Shannon asked me if I could do it, I said "100, 93, 86, 79, 72, 65, 58, 51, 44, 37, 30, 23, 16, 9, 2." It took maybe fifteen seconds.

Shannon said "Wow." And we drove in silence for an hour.

"What an asshole, I am" I thought. How infinitely more kind to say "Hell, no I can't. No one can. That's the most unfair question I've ever heard. They cannot possibly make a diagnosis based on the answer to that." That's what I should have said... but I did not, and I

will never forgive myself. Sometimes, you only get one chance to do the right thing. Legan's Law 4.

Further Digression

Shannon and I were speaking by telephone with one of her (many) psychiatrists. This was something about which we sometimes argued. Shannon was constantly wanting a new psychiatrist, therapist, or counselor. And she had many. I did not understand. She was physically ill, not mentally ill, I thought. But I played along. Why deny her this? There was no expense and no harm done. During that conversation I expressed my frustration with the professionals being unable to deliver an objective diagnosis, instead of the subjective diagnosis upon which we were placing our trust.

His reply was one of the best answers to any question I have ever heard. He said, "I understand your point, and I think of it often myself. We have now monitored over a million patients with this disease, patients who we have confirmed through autopsy" (they find the Lewy Bodies within the brain) "and we monitor about one hundred data points on each. That's a swarm of one hundred million bits of data. That amount of data approaches objectivity."

Holy smoke, what did he just say? He said, though gently stated, that our situation is hopeless, without uttering those words. Having watched as Shannon's symptoms worsened as predicted by the playbook, I knew that he was correct.

November 2, 2021

Today, we will go to Hot Springs. Shannon needs a haircut, and I have an eye exam in anticipation of cataract surgery, which I plan to delay until 2022... just too many holiday details to complicate with a ten doctor visit project of dual eye surgery. So, today's appointments overlap in time... driving Shannon absolutely crazy with concern and confusion. In two days, she has a hair coloring appointment. Then, the following day, we will drive to her daughter's home in Jackson, MS, before driving to Baton Rouge for an LSU football game on Saturday. Shannon is unable to walk through Dillard's without stopping to rest her back, and I am dreading the walk from the car to our seats at the stadium. Shannon's daughter, Bev, is a wonderful daughter and a very intelligent woman... a PhD therapist specializing in eating disorders. She wants to do something, anything, for her mom. I get that. She had planned a mother/daughter trip to Napa Valley, CA, for the first of December, but wisely canceled it after realizing the difficulty surrounding Shannon's mobility. I tried to convince Bev to cancel this football trip, but she would not. She has not yet seen Shannon's mobility difficulties in person, but she will see it this weekend. If this trip is as complicated and draining for Shannon as I fear, the next one will not come to a vote... I will simply pull rank and make the decision. My genuine concern is not just that it might be a challenging trip. My concern is that it could be very trying and painful for Shannon... and that an experience like that might be a setback... pushing Shannon's disease (or at least its manifestations) faster than they might otherwise progress. In the interest of full disclosure, I should mention that heart problems have me worried about my ability to walk a mile to the stadium and then climb into the heavens for my seat.

Following the trip, which will take either three or four days, we are planning for a big Thanksgiving. We've rented a nearby VRBO house for the weekend. Bev and her husband will stay there (along with Battle, the German Shorthaired Pointer), and Shannon's son Brad, from Arizona, who hopes to come and bring his son Benson (Shannon's grandson) along. My son Dave is coming, hopefully with his girlfriend. I have a Turducken in the fridge, and I'll add a standing rib roast if necessary... probably will not be since there are vegans among the guests.

I think that brings me up to date on this diary. I'll try to keep it current.

Digression

I have been undergoing treatment for a heart ailment, left ventricular hypertrophy, for over a year. This is a condition wherein an essential heart muscle has become hard and oversized (probably due to years of inadequately treated high blood pressure) and is, therefore, unable to deliver enough oxygenated blood to wherever it needs to go. Shortness of breath is the result, and I have that issue constantly. I ran a half marathon at age fifty, and now I cannot walk to the mailbox without stopping to catch my breath. The loss of stamina simply pisses me off. I take pills to make me pee, pills to lower my blood pressure, pills to calm me down, pills to help my kidneys, pills, and more pills. (Nothing like Shannon, who takes over twenty per day, but still emasculating in a strange sort of way.)

November 11, 2021

Yesterday was a good day. Shannon got her hair cut while I went to the eye doctor. Her cut was over before I could return to pick her up, and she did not panic. Instead, she went to a Mexican restaurant next door and had a Margarita while waiting. Encouraging. Hair looks good, too. Today, we return to Hot Springs, and I will run errands while she gets her hair colored. We will see.

November 18, 2021

We went to watch LSU play Arkansas last weekend. We drove to Jackson on Friday and spent the night with Bev and her husband. Then, we drove to a VRBO home about 40 miles east of Baton Rouge before leaving midafternoon for the 6:30 game at Tiger Stadium. IT WAS MISERABLE.

It was cold. We parked a half mile from the stadium and rode a bicycle-taxi-rickshaw to the stadium. Sixty bucks to park, sixty more to ride to the stadium, sixty more to return to the car. Which we did before half-time. Upon arriving at the stadium, we had to trudge up six or so ramp levels, then about twenty flights of stairs. It was probably equal to thirty flights of stairs, and I was out of breath and unwilling to push any further. Shannon, on the other hand, handled it like a U.S. Marine. As we approached our ticketed seats, it became obvious that our seats were at the very top of the stadium. It was also obvious that many seats were unfilled and would stay that way – right where we already were - about fifty steps lower than our reserved seats. It was an inconsequential game, it was cold, and many ticket holders were not going to show up. So, I suggested that we sit a little lower, not in the seats for which we had tickets (which were flat metal benches) but in the plastic molded seats we had already reached – so that I would not have to climb any higher. There were hundreds of them empty. But Bev's husband said, “Let’s go find our seats, we can come back,” and I stayed behind as he, Bev, and Shannon continued upward to the cold, flat metal seats. They did not return. I thought, until near kickoff, that they were watching to see if latecomers would fill the more comfortable empty seats... but no one did. Yet, they did not come down to join me, and by game time, I felt truly alone and deserted. Before halftime, after sitting on those miserable seats, they were ready to leave and actually descended past me, still sitting there by myself and VERY pissed off. My own wife had followed Bev’s husband to those miserable seats, and never even checked on me. And now she was leaving without checking on me. I was heartbroken and quite angry... unwilling to spend another second with Bev and her husband. When we returned to the VRBO, I told them that I was driving home immediately, and after a bit of quarreling, Shannon got into the car with me, and we drove all night... over 600 miles... to our Arkansas home. I know that she is going to become more and more belligerent. I expect that. But she is so thoughtless... so unsupportive even now... even before the disease progresses, that I am frankly amazed. I would expect her to at least recognize the responsibility that she places on me. At least be on my side most of the time. But it seems that she never is. If I was unjustly accused of a crime, I am certain that she would assume I was guilty. And that is just the way that it is gonna be until this thing runs its course. It was already set up to be the toughest thing of my life, and now it appears that I will be totally alone and unappreciated as I do it.

Shannon is constantly depressed and cries a lot. She talks about suicide. I've kept a 38-caliber pistol in the master bedroom nightstand for years, and I removed it. I took her to Walmart and Lowe's today, and she was confused at both. Not nearly as energetic as she had been at the game, she sat down at every opportunity, limped, shuffled about, and was negative about everything. Man, this is getting harder by the day.

November 20, 2021

I bought a new TV- a 70 inch - which is huge. I moved the den TV, which is about 60 inches, to my bedroom. So, the enormous TV was delivered on Wednesday, and I couldn't get it working. Suddenlink customer service couldn't help me, despite two long phone calls. So, the technician came today and got it going in less than 5 minutes. Then, we had to get that huge thing on our TV cabinet, which is too short for the TV legs to fit. We shopped for a replacement cabinet. Something longer. But a good one was $350, and we found nothing at the second-hand shops that would work. I decided to mount the TV on a board, 60" X 16", and then sit the board on the existing cabinet. The legs were to be affixed to the board with zip ties. So, I enlisted Shannon in the project and she was a great helper. She only complained a little, was generally supportive, and had some good ideas. It was a nice husband/wife project and it reminded me of the fun times we had in the motor home. The TV is wonderful. It fills the room and has a picture that literally shows the blades of grass on a football field. Shannon was curious as to why I wanted it. Well, the TV in my bedroom was failing sporadically and appeared to be headed for the scrap heap. That was my excuse. But the real reason is that I think TV will be an ever-increasing part of my life for about 5 years. We might as well try to enjoy it.

Tomorrow morning, we drive to Shreveport to see the home where Patricia Hayes grew up. Her father, Mr. Nelson, is staying at her and Gary's home as he spirals toward death, and the old homestead is for sale. But it is in terrible shape and needs a lot of work before being marketed, and I am the "expert" at that. So, we leave at 8AM, meet Gary and Patricia at the house at noon, spend two hours there, and then drive home. Shannon was a little bitchy about going, but I explained that Gary and Patricia had given me a ton of business in 2013, and had been friends since 1966, and that I simply owed it to them. So, tonight, we both went to bed at 7PM, but I awoke at 10PM and wrote this. Sleep is not my friend, lately.

December 1, 2021

What a Thanksgiving week. Daughter Bev, her husband, and Battle (the dog) picked up son Brad at the Little Rock airport and arrived at Hot Springs Village about midnight Wednesday. My son Dave arrived two hours earlier. We talked and drank until 2AM and then they checked into their VRBO. I went to bed and was up and cooking by 9AM.

I've cooked many Thanksgiving meals, but this was among the toughest. Overdid everything. Too much of everything. Shannon tried to help but was just in the way. Others also tried to help, but... well, you know how it is. Somewhat surprisingly, Bev's husband was the best kitchen helper imaginable. He is one of those people who pays attention and anticipates what the cook might do next. The following day was Taco Night - more work. And the next day was a full omelet breakfast for everyone.

It was a long and frankly miserable weekend only because of the work, not the company. Shannon was able to see both of her children together, in the same room. That is an incredible gift to an aging parent, believe me, I know. I was thrilled to have provided her with that opportunity.

Her son-in-law is a piece of work. He is an attorney, and apparently quite successful. He is one of those guys who interrupts, a lot. We were gathered in the den, and he went to relieve himself as Brad was telling a story. When he returned to the room, he loudly proclaimed his reappearance, said something unimportant, then told Brad, "Go ahead and finish your story… I'm sorry to interrupt." And this was not a single interruption; it was part of a pattern with which I had become quite annoyed.

So, in a sample of inhospitality worthy of a chapter by Emily Post, I asked, "Then, why did you? Why did you interrupt?"

The room fell silent. Brad stared at his shoes. Shannon gave me that look. My son David looked as if he had swallowed a pineapple.

Charging into the awkward silence, I said to everyone, "Look, this is not his normal behavior. He does not want to be the guy who interrupts. That is not him. I simply think he ought to be reminded."

Silence. I was clearly an asshole. What else is new?

Today, we went to UAMS to meet with Shannon's PCP, Dr. Hassan. He confirmed the terminality of Shannon's illness and called in a social worker to talk with us. Not much help there. She seemed more concerned about me than about Shannon. She was a very prim and proper woman of about our age and asked if I was holding up well. And what did I want from this experience? It was an innocent question, but I was somehow annoyed by it.

I bowed up and told her, "Look at my eyes. I am the toughest motherfucker in this building. There is nothing in the world that I cannot do... that I will not do... when I set my mind to it. So, I am frustrated as all hell to be in a life-and-death situation where I have NO CONTROL AT ALL. Yes, I'm hurting, but I'll be okay. And the ONLY thing that I want now, besides a miracle, is to be able to look back someday and say, 'I did my best.'" Shannon and I went to dinner in Little Rock and arrived home well after dark. Short days, but long nights.

December 8, 2021

Went to Little Rock again today to see Shannon's neurologist. She added a dopamine replacement drug to the ELEVEN that Shannon takes now. LBD is characterized by mood swings like a roller coaster. We are on the high side of that ride now and for the last few days. So, Shannon had a good day, almost like old times. She's sleeping comfortably now, and I'm probably headed for another night of sleepless worrying.

Chapter 4
2022
Any Chance, Any Cost

I've grown used to losing what I'm fondest of.
"Someone Like You"- Bob McDill and Dickie Lee as sung by Emmy Lou Harris

January 14, 2022

Shannon is doing well. Better than I expected. She and I, however, are doing very poorly. I have learned that I cannot expect her to take my side in any situation, and I have not been able to accept that. But I must accept it. At least I can now attribute this odd behavior to her illness, which I have done. I have decided that it is my purpose, for as long as I am allowed, to make her comfortable in every way I can and squeeze my own feelings into a spot deep down from which they may someday be rescued. I reached a tipping point, of sorts. Right now, it is all about Shannon.

Digression

A real estate broker holds in his hands a great part of the future of the sales associates who work under his (or her, of course) broker's license. The associate must be confident that the broker will back the associate if there is an argument about a broken rule or ethical standard or (especially) the proper disbursement of a commission payment. I supervised, trained, and managed hundreds of real estate salespeople during my thirty-five-year career, and I understood this from a personal and business viewpoint. So, I said to each batch of aspiring agents:

"I am on your side. EVERY time. If I walk into a bar, and find you in a barfight, I will not ask, "Who started it" or "Who is at fault?"

"I will pick up a chair and start swinging it. Now, if I find out later that you insulted the bartender and flushed his wife's head in the toilet, we will have to talk." The associates always laughed at that, but it is surprising how often a broker is required to fight for his agents. So, that is my mentality when supporting a friend. In for a penny, in for a pound.

All of that to get to Tibby. A friend of mine since third grade, and of Shannon's since tenth, Tibby is tall, boisterous, opinionated, and loud. And I had loved her since we met. She was one of maybe ten people in the world that I called a "friend," and we were, of course, friends on Facebook. So, Tibby became very angry about some of my comments opposing Donald Trump, and she un-friended me! I was speechless at the time but forgot about it. Maybe a year later, Tibby messaged me, apologized, and asked me to please re-friend her. "I'll get over it," I said and complied. It wasn't a big deal to me... until she un-friended me AGAIN. I was bursting with anger and told Shannon about it.

Shannon then phoned Tibby and talked with her as an old friend, before telling me she had done so. To say that I was angry would vastly understate my reaction! I told Shannon, "If someone did that to you, I would call them out and denounce them in righteous indignation. I would rise with my sword and smite them. NO ONE could ever screw with you without screwing with me!"

Shannon said she wanted to leave this world with folks thinking positively about her. We argued in the strongest of terms, and that was before the football game in Baton Rouge when I went insane with anger. In the end, I did nothing, of course. I blamed it on the disease and moved on. A terminal illness gives one an explanation for the otherwise inexplicable.

February 16, 2022

Watching Shannon's decline is like watching a train wreck in slow motion. And it's like watching it for the tenth time. Though I am seeing it for the first time, I've read so much and studied the probable path of the disease so much that it all seems familiar. This paragraph is prompted by an episode that happened on Saturday ten days ago, and some following events.

Shannon came to me that morning, much earlier than her usual 11AM wake-up. Apparently, she had not slept at all, which is common for me but not her. She was more anxious than I have seen her – ever. She asked for one of my clonazepam pills, a mild sedative, and I gave her half of one. As she began to calm down, she related to me that she had seen hallucinations all night long. She asked, "Where is Brad." "Is Bev taking him to the airport" "How are we going to feed all these people?" We were, of course, alone. When the pill took effect, she went to sleep. I stayed with her the entire day, reading in bed as she slept fitfully beside me. She woke, at least halfway, again and again. Always asking the same questions about Brad, Bev, and Bryan. It was excruciating for me. When she woke more fully, LATE in the afternoon, she continued to ask those same questions. At one point, she turned her head quickly and said, "Did you see that?" What? I asked. "That little boy who just walked into the bathroom."

I related these events to Bev, and she phoned Shannon. When Shannon asked me, while talking to Bev, "What pill was that" I KNEW that I was certain to hear more about it. Bev made far less of it than I expected. To her credit, she did not chastise me for giving Shannon an unprescribed med. However, knowing that Shannon had been groggy from that half-pill caused Bev and Brad to question my judgment about the hallucinations. Now, I understand that. They do not see her often. They do not see the decline as I do. When they do see her, their presence supercharges Shannon's mental state… she is so happy to see them that her mood obscures the pain and confusion that clouds every day that she is with me. Shannon loves me - or at least the thought of me - of that, I have no doubt. But I am not in the same league with her own kids, nor should I be. I understand that, too. When Shannon is not with them, she talks to them by phone (especially Bev), often daily. You know how phone calls are. Information is skipped or lost in translation, questions are answered more simply, and details are missed. So, both Bev and Brad questioned the hallucinations, and why wouldn't they? After all, she is their mom, and they want to find some way to believe that she is not really as sick as the doctors say, and there are days when she does not seem that sick. Some days, she seems like the same ditzy blonde that I came to love. The same one who piloted a thirty-five-foot-long motorhome through the treacherous mountains of Oregon without ever putting a wheel wrong, but who slipped ever so gradually; so gradually that I did not take enough notice though we slept in the same bed. Slipped so far that she could not count the change in a cash register. Damn! I even thought she was faking some of it. Or at least not trying hard enough. Then, she started hitting things with the car, once driving through a three-foot swale and into our front yard. She became afraid of everything. And I still took it less seriously than I should have. So, it's not realistic to expect her kids to accept her declining condition. They are not watching it daily, they want her to be OK, and they want to maintain hope. That's the worst part of this disease. The hopelessness. Damn, even with terminal cancer, there is hope. Not here.

So, last night, we had a ZOOM call. The four of us. Shannon was terrified before the call. She is so afraid that she will end up in a nursing home like her mom, slumped in a wheelchair, drooling on a bib. That will not happen to Shannon if I am alive to prevent it. If I am gone, Bev and Brad will take those reins, I'm sure of it. Shannon has talked of assisted suicide, and we tried, the three of us, to explain how that simply cannot happen. Even if we wanted to help her do it, there are so many legal restrictions that it cannot be accomplished. Shannon said she understood, but I am certain she did not accept it. I have hidden my revolver, and she could not load the .22, so I feel safe there. After talking with her kids, and after I stood my ground about the clonazepam, I think we are all on the same page. Brad has shown more compassion than I knew he had, and Bev is doing a lot to help.

One of the purposes of last night's call was to get everyone on the same page about Shannon's future care. My position on that has not changed, and I repeated it. I'll take care of her, here in this house… our home… her home… as long as I am able, until I cannot keep her safe and assist adequately with her hygiene. At that point, if I need help, we will hire live-in assistance. I feel confident that I can find the right person. Someone with nursing or home care skills, and who needs room and board. I can bring her in and give her a place to stay, food to eat, wine to drink, a TV to watch, and a small salary. For that, I expect the assistant to help with Shannon's personal care. Bathing, ass wiping, makeup - everything that I cannot do or that I would not want a spouse to do for me if the situation was reversed. When Shannon's condition worsens to a point beyond that level of help, I'll call on Medicaid for long-term assistance. As I write this, the financial actions necessary to make that work are in progress.

I promised some weeks ago to be more kind to Shannon, and I have kept that promise. Within reason, and within my ability to provide, she gets everything she wants or asks for. If she says let's go out to dinner, I get dressed, and if she then says that she needs a nap, I do not get upset or take it personally. She is NOT trying to be difficult, and I take it all in stride. That was tough at first, but not now.

We have been laughing a lot lately. Laughing at the silly stuff that makes good friends laugh. A few days ago, we were trying, the two of us, to stuff a huge blanket into a storage bag. We made it look like a scene from I Love Lucy. We collapsed on the floor, laughing until we cried. That has happened a couple of times lately. In the motorhome, it happened frequently. Once, while lying in bed at Half Moon Bay, CA, I watched as Buddy simply attacked the carpeted floor. Scratching with both front paws, like he was digging a hole – he was quite serious. I told Shannon, "Look at him… he's working at that as if we are paying him." Well, that got Shannon going. She said, "We need to get him a hard hat and a lunch box" to go with his new worker image. And that image caused us to laugh like children… Foreman Buddy… it still does. Damn, I miss that, and I am really going to miss the life we should be allowed.

Time for me to put this away. A real estate appraiser is coming in an hour to inspect the house. This is part of the process of getting a reverse mortgage, which will mean THAT WE NEVER AGAIN OWE A MORTGAGE PAYMENT! That is just one of the financial moves I am making to allow Shannon and me some peace of mind as her disease progresses.

March 26, 2022 - 6:02 AM

I did not go to bed tonight, sleeping is getting more difficult. Shannon had a bad night Thursday and came into the den asking who had been knocking on her window. Whomever it had been asked her, "Where did you take my yellow moo-moo?" More hallucinations. I am going to change the locks on the front and garage doors, then add some kind of security device to the sliding glass door to the deck. Fear of her sleepwalking. This is getting very real.

Thursday was a tough day for me. Sold the Yamaha after riding it over thirty thousand miles in the last six years. It brought almost four thousand dollars, so I now have 50 one-hundred-dollar bills hidden in the house. Working on getting 300 of them. Gonna need cash, that no one knows I have, someday, probably within two years.

We have a busy spring planned. Besides the usual cluster of doctor visits, there will be a trip to Austin on April 8th-12th for my son Hank's bachelor party weekend, and a trip to the Mayo Clinic in Rochester, Minnesota, in late April. Then, Hank's wedding AND college graduation, Austin again, in mid-May.

The Mayo Clinic visit deserves a paragraph or two. Shannon worked on this alone, totally without my help. She contacted them, communicated with them, and presented them with the required insurance information. (How can this woman be dying?) And they agreed to see her and review her case. Of course, no one could take issue with reaching for the best medical advice available. If there is ANY chance that the diagnosis is incorrect, if there is any chance that we are treating the wrong disease, we must take this trip. Any chance, any cost.

But there is a risk in going. What if her diagnosis is confirmed? That would essentially be the best doctors in the nation announcing, "You are going to die soon." So, the hopelessness would become even greater. I am terrified of that, and I believe it to be the likeliest scenario.

We went to Hot Springs today. Bought some clothes and groceries. Lunch at a deli. I am getting Shannon out of the house every day.

Even if I have to cajole and shame her, I am relentless. Maybe just Sonic for cheese sticks. Sometimes more. After selling the motorcycle, we celebrated with drinks and appetizers at the Sand Trap Bar and Grill. I want to believe that activity… any activity… is good for her. I think I probably believe this because it offers something that I can do. "Hey, look. I'm taking her out for lunch." Simply getting dressed and into the car is good for her. Working on a crossword is good for her. Going for a walk is good for her.

I already miss that motorcycle. I'll miss Shannon. I miss our past life, even now.

I'm gonna try to get a little sleep now.

April 4, 2022

Shannon got a "cold" yesterday. She thinks it's covid, or the flu, and sent me to Walgreens for a covid test, which they don't sell, and decongestants, which they do. She says that she has a fever and wants to go to see her doctor in Little Rock today. She also sees a group of kids playing in the house and does not know whether it is now 10AM or 10PM. Last night, I stayed in the recliner until about 4AM, guarding against her sleepwalking. Usually, I can sleep from about 4 to about 9. But this morning at 5:45AM, as I was asleep, Shannon was hunting for me in the house and loudly called out my name from the hallway. Her shout startled me awake, and it took several minutes for my heart rate to return to normal. I guided her back to bed, but she wanted to leave the TV on so loud that I couldn't sleep. I returned to the recliner and grabbed a nap. The plumber came at 10AM for some minor repairs, so that was that. While he was working in her bathroom and Shannon was safe and napping in my bedroom, she again got out of bed and came hunting for me. Have you called the doctor? Will you call the doctor? We have the drive-through Covid test scheduled for noon. This is about the fifth time Shannon has contracted a sniffle, and her thoughts immediately jumped straight to covid. I am afraid that much more of this is in store.

Last night, I called Hank and told him I could not attend his "bachelor weekend," scheduled for this week. I have too much to do and too many things to think about. If he was disappointed, he hid it well, and we talked for half an hour. Then Dave called, and WE talked for half an hour. I wish I could go. I want to be there for Hank, but my back hurts when I walk, so I can't play golf with Hank and his friends, and I doubt that I could walk from the parking lot to the grandstand at the Moto GP race on Sunday. I am very disappointed. The procedure on my sciatic back has been, to this point, a failure. Dr. Rosenzweig will repeat it in two weeks. It is the diagnostic procedure for determining which nerve is causing the pain, before deadening it. During the time when he wants to do that, we will be at the Mayo Clinic. So, a delay there.

Digression

Caretakers are often advised to take care of themselves. There's a lot of sleeplessness, stress, and frustration. A common concern is that caretakers may ignore their own health issues or self-care because they need the time to take care of their charge. Apparently, there are many patients who outlive their caretakers. I suppose there is something to that, but there's more, I am convinced. I think at least some of the dead caregivers were just old folks, many as old as the patient. Damn, I am 72 years old as I write this in 2022. If I were to die before Shannon, you could not possibly blame my death on caretaking stress. You would blame it on the fact that I am a hard-living, heavy-drinking 72-year-old old fart who simply reached his "sell-by" date.

Do you remember the Ogden Nash poem "Old Men?"

Old Men

People expect old men to die,
They do not really mourn old men.
Old men are different. People look
At them with eyes that wonder when...
People watch with unshocked eyes;
But the old men know when an old man dies.

April 5, 2022

Shannon and I have covid. She was tested at noon yesterday, and I began to feel crappy as the day wore on. So, her test is positive, and mine is set for 11 AM today. I'm certain that it will be positive, too, though her symptoms are far worse than mine. Last Saturday, before she showed any symptoms, I had a "shortness of breath" spell and took a few whiffs of oxygen from a bottle of Boost. That hasn't been necessary since 2020. Now I know why I needed a sniff.

If Shannon is not a lot better tomorrow, we will take her to a doctor and maybe even a hospital. In fact, we will probably be required to go to an emergency room because she might not allowed into a regular clinic. It's going to be a hassle, but what isn't these days?

April 9, 2022

As promised, we went to the ER and departed six hours later with a scrip for anti-virals. I was so annoyed with Shannon. Her voice was little more than a squeak for two days, but when the doctor showed up, she suddenly became "Chatty Cathy," speaking clearly and even joking. Aaarrggg. This is a terrible thing, this LBD. Its ups and downs are SO frustrating.

A half hour ago, at 3:00 AM, she lumbered into the den where I was watching a PBS program about Alzheimer's caregivers, and asked, "Where are they?" gesturing around the house.

"Who?" I ask.

"Patti and Bev," she answers. Patti died two years ago, and Bev is sleeping in Jackson.

"You've been dreaming," I say, as gently as possible. She dropped her head and shuffled back to bed, clearly more frustrated than I was. This is hard on me, but infinitely harder on her. It's not physically painful, though that stage might come. Still, I try to imagine what it would be like to have moments of complete lucidity, and, in those moments, to realize, like awakening from a dream, that this really is your life. What a horrible sentence, and understanding it just makes it much worse.

My first covid test was negative, and I knew it was wrong. But it allowed me to go grocery shopping in good conscience and get the Acura's rear end repaired. I backed into a pickup truck a couple of weeks ago. The body shop ordered and painted the valence, and I waited on their front porch bench, eating a tuna roll, for the hour and a half it took to install the freshly painted piece.

I tested again, and it was positive. My PCP called in some meds, and now, two days later, I feel quite good… though I am gonna fake it through this weekend, the weekend of The Masters and the Moto GP race at Circuit of the Americas in Austin, on TV. I should be there. This is Hank's "bachelor weekend." His cousins, brother Dave, and some friends will drink too much, listen to too much country rock, and have too much fun. I dropped out, even before the Covid thing. I was foolish to agree to go because it presented the problem of what I should do with Shannon. Sunday, we would have gone to the race. I feared the walk from the car to the grandstands, Shannon would have been even more miserable than normal, and Hank and Dave would have felt obligated to go with me. Oh, they would have gone (against their wills) because they would have thought it necessary. "One more race, about which we know nothing, for Pop's sake," they would have thought. That whole thing did not sound like fun, and I dropped out the day before we found out about Covid. If I had waited just one day, I would have had the perfect excuse to stay home. So, I vacillated over the decision before making the call to Hank. He was gracious, calling it a "big ask" to invite me. He realized it was a 900-mile round trip, with a repeat in May for the wedding. So, he took it like the man he has become. I just wish I had waited one day; there is nothing like having a perfect excuse when you do not want to do something.

Last night, I watched a PBS documentary about a man's descent into bipolar depression. It was written, filmed in large measure, and produced by the man's sister, Sandra Luckow, who I found out later is a well-known and award-winning documentarian. I messaged to her FB account:

> "Greetings from Hot Springs Village, Arkansas
>
> I just watched the PBS documentary about your brother, Duane, "That Way Madness Lies." Even knowing that a FB message was unlikely to reach you, I felt compelled to write to compliment your extraordinary work and even more to remark upon the commitment that you have shown to your family. The patience, self-control, and devotion that you display in this film are inspiring. I did not realize, while watching, that you are so well awarded, educated, and credentialed in this art. But the more I watched, the more I realized the level of professionalism; thus, I was unsurprised to learn that you are an artist.
>
> As have many people, I experienced a wee bit of the experiences you document. I reached my end far quicker than you. Upon my parents'

> death, and after investing hundreds of thousands of dollars and every emotional cent that I had in the piggy bank, I gave up on my sister. The bough broke when I received one last call from a social worker who said, "You have to come get her. You have to handle this." I told her simply that I did not have to, and that I wouldn't. I had realized that my sister was not my problem. I was my problem.
>
> David Legan,
>
> PS. In googling you, I discovered that your film has received many awards and was shown at the Hot Springs International Women's Film Festival just a month ago. I live 25 miles from that theater, and I am so annoyed with myself for not seeing it there. Did not even know of the event."

She replied immediately, gracious and seemingly honored by the compliments.

> "David, Rest assured that I did receive your touching note and it means so much to me. The hope that this might be relatable to other people and help them to understand that their own experience was not isolated but part of a much larger world. Best, Sandra"

Gonna wrap it up for the night/morning/whatever you call it when it's 4AM and you are still awake. Maybe I will finish that television program about caregivers. Gruesome stuff.

April 25, 2022 - 4:12AM

Covid sort of knocked the crap out of both of us. It began around April 5 and continued through my birthday on April 13 and into the following week… about the 20th. Charlie was here from the 11th through the 15th, and he did not get sick... probably because he had the virus a year ago and he is vaccinated. Shannon and I are grateful for the vax and booster… our symptoms were mild but still crappy. I think I was exposed to Covid at Springhill Surgical Center, where Dr. Rosenzweig gave me some injections to determine if he could fix my back with his nerve-deadening needle.

We should be in Rochester, Minnesota right now, as I write this, awaiting Shannon's first tests at the Mayo Clinic. They messaged us on Thursday, with only one day remaining before travel, to say that they had not even applied to the insurance company for $15,000 in tests. Did we want to guarantee that amount, personally? Well, not really. So, we re-scheduled it for mid-July. Maybe for the best. We are still wrung out from Covid and sleeping about 18 hours a day.

This morning, Shannon said, "I feel GREAT." What a wonderful sound that was. So, we went into Benton. She shopped at Target and then Home Depot, where I made the mistake of letting her out of my sight. She panicked a bit… lost in the garden section of Home Depot. I was fifty yards away in the car, and quickly retrieved her. But it taught me not to do that again. Tonight, she burst into tears again. She is doing this often. Her words are frequently similar. "You did not sign up for this. It should not be your job to take care of me. I do not want to be a burden. Why is this happening to me?" But tonight, she added, "Have you and Bev looked into long-term care for me?"

Well, Bev and I have not, but I have. I am gathering information, and, perhaps more importantly, cash. I think that Shannon will need long-term full-time care within three years, maybe less. That means Medicaid. I want her to stay in this house for as long as possible. I am also hoping for help from Medicaid with her at-home caretaking.

So far, she is having no trouble with her hygiene and self-care. Every Saturday, we sit in her bed and sort pills. There are about fifteen for the mornings, another ten for late afternoon, and three or four for bedtime. So, we sort them into three different "Monday-Sunday" trays – morning, noon, and night. It takes about an hour, sitting side by side, squabbling over how many of each we need. Shannon always becomes confused. There is simply no way she could do this alone. But together, we worked out a system, and it's something we can do together.

There is a woman in Hot Springs, Mrs. Rogers, whose husband died of LBD in 2021. She is trying to form a support group for LBD caregivers. She is very pleasant and always willing to talk with me, but in six months, she has found only me to go to the group meetings, so there have been none. I would certainly attend, even if there was only one other attendee. After watching TV programs about caregivers, and reading a lot, I still do not know what to expect. I need "benchmarks" of the progression of the disease. I need to know what to expect. I need to speak with others who have experience.

There is no damned way to find answers to many questions, and almost all questions lead back to time. I spoke to Mrs. Rogers for about an hour last Friday. Her husband lapsed into a permanent hallucination after watching his beloved St. Louis Cardinals on TV and imagined that he was playing second base. One night, after a televised Cardinal game, he said, "I'm going to bed now, gotta rest, playing second base for the Cardinals tomorrow." Those were the last words he spoke. He was noncommunicative the next day, lingered for 72 hours, and died. I asked, as gently as possible, what was the cause of death. "His mind shut down… he forgot how to breathe… his heart forgot to beat." He had been ill for nine years. In Shannon's case, nine years would run from 2015 to 2024. That is scary. From first symptoms to death, nine years. He had suffered an "event" more than a decade before the diagnosis. She emphasized, over and over, the up-and-down nature of this disease. I have read this many times and concluded that there are no benchmarks. No predictability. No hope, no measure, no expectations. So, my preparations are:

1. Accumulate cash and articles that convert easily - guns and guitars, for example.
2. Ensure that Shannon does not have significant cash in her account… not more than two thousand dollars.
3. Reduce expenses and save as much as possible.
4. Monitor her meds like an owl watching a mouse.
5. Keep her as active as possible.

Mrs. Rogers had "hospice care" help for several years, paid for by Medicaid. Hospice caregivers, three times a week, two hours at a time. Gave him a bath and gave her time to go shopping. That amount of assistance will not be enough for us. If I were given a two-hour break at this moment, I would sleep for an hour and fifty-nine minutes. And I cannot imagine taking care of Shannon's hygiene. So, I hope to employ as much hospice care as the system will allow and hire much more. Possibly even a live-in assistant.

Digression

Mike was my partner in the real estate business. He is worthy of his own book, but ...well, not now. After he died in 2004, I closed our company in 2005. I took some time off, then signed with Diamond Realty in Bossier City (Shreveport's sister city, across the Red River.) The owner is Travis Hargrave. I was the only other person in the office who knew what he was dealing with. Only I knew his job, and because of that, for a while, we were friends – well, close. Not close friends, just close to being friends.

On my second day there, his partner called me, preening for a "stockholders fight," and asked me to manage the company if he won. Every company needs a "sponsoring broker" and he wanted that to be me. He knew I had a Broker's license, and a mutual acquaintance recommended me. After meeting with him and his wife at Waffle

House, I asked him if I could try to settle his dispute with Travis. And, then I did it. I mediated their dispute, drafted an agrement that he and Travis signed, and a disrupting fight over ownership was avoided. Travis told me later that his attorney was miffed. He had wanted to settle their disagreement himself.

Travis named me "Diamond of the Month" early on, and I was getting a start on selling a few houses. Almost anything would be better than the exhausting duties as a brokerage manager, which had driven me into depression only five years before.

Travis came to me sometime in 2010 and asked me, "Do you know much about property management?"

"Well, heck yes, I do. That was all I did from 1996 until Mike died in 2004."

"Would you consider being a property manager for Diamond?"

"Yes, I would consider that."

The negotiations that we conducted and the agreement we reached are not the subject of this book, so I will not belabor them. It is enough to say that I created his property management division, managed it for a couple of years, and received $4,000 per month, every month from 2012 through 2018.

This was my retirement. It had funded our motorhome adventures and our life in Hot Springs Village. He missed only a few payments, with the unpaid balance approaching $20,000 by 2024, when he stopped paying altogether. In addition to the burden of caring for Shannon, I then had to do it alone with a failing heart and much less money. We had a genuine crisis on our hands.

May 2, 2022

Friday afternoon, I drove Shannon to Ruston, Louisiana, to meet Bev so that Shannon could spend the weekend with her in Jackson. I had an injection procedure in the early morning. Then we headed south from Little Rock, Shannon driving as I emerged from the anesthesia. We met Bev at about 5PM, then I drove straight back, stayed awake all night, and finally went to sleep after sun-up. Then, Saturday night, another insomnia, another 7AM bedtime. Shannon woke me with a phone call two hours later, and again at 11AM. Her feet were swollen, and she wanted to come home. Everyone wants to be at home when ailing. Though sleepless, I understood and left home early Sunday afternoon and drove to Ruston, retrieved Shannon, and drove her home. She went straight to her bedroom and, except for two trips to the kitchen, has been there since. That's about 17 hours of the last 18. She spends more and more time there. I try to get her out of the house, or at least dressed, every day, but even that is becoming difficult.

Her friend Dawn and husband Eric are coming for a weekend visit. Shannon is already worried about cleaning the house. They are pulling a camper and will park it in the front yard front. She's worried about that, too.

May 20, 2022

Shannon's friends came for a two-night stay, and we had a good time. Shannon, as usual, was energized by her friends and enjoyed every minute.

Last weekend, we drove to Austin for Hank's graduation and wedding weekend. It was a great time, hobbled only by my preference to be at home. We stayed with John Haigler, in Tyler, Texas on the way down.

It is always great to see John, a friend since 1972. But his guest bed sucks, and I slept on the couch.

We finished the drive the next day, checked into a $300-a-night hotel, and had lunch with Hank that afternoon. Shannon seemed great… actually better than me… for the entire trip. I get SO short of breath, so easily. I cannot walk from the room to the bar without a stop to a rest.

Hank's graduation was a gas. The grads have a tradition of jumping into the San Marcos River, directly beside the Auditorium, in full cap and gown, and Hank did not disappoint- doing a perfect 360 backflip into the water. Later that evening, we went to a pre-wedding party at a VRBO he and Mandy had rented for the occasion. I paid for the pizza and drinks.

Now would be a good time to write about Mandy Mendez (and now) Legan. She is precious. Tall and thin, high class, high intelligence, and a marvelous sense of humor, fashion and humanity. Beautiful, vegan like Hank, rock-climber like Hank, driven like Hank. She specializes in fundraising for non-profit organizations and accepted a position with Tony Hawk's skateboard park initiative. They build playgrounds in underserved urban areas. She works 100% remotely, and their upcoming move to Denver, where Hank will attend law school, is a non-event for her working life.

The wedding was a marvelous affair. Planned 100% by Mandy, it took place on a "party barge" on the San Gabriel River. It was held at sundown, with the city lights of Austin glowing in the background and a beautiful Texas sunset accenting the occasion. I was particularly impressed by their friends. A more mature and kinder group of young folks I have never met. Many of them stopped by to introduce themselves to Shannon and me, all with the politeness of diplomats and the clear-eyed confidence of a Christian holding four aces.

We drove home after the wedding. A little over five hundred miles without so much as a hiccup. We arrived home after midnight to find our A/C unit had failed. It has now been almost a week, and the warranty company has shipped the unit. Even with the warranty, our cost is still about two grand. When I told Shannon about that cost, she said, “I am so glad that you did the things necessary to put us in a position to pay that without hardship.” That comment made me feel great.

My old friend Lyn Anderson arrived today for a short visit. We now agree on nothing regarding religion and politics, but I love him just the same. We went to the Oaklawn Casino to see Don McLean perform. There was a LOT of gray hair in that audience. Bye, bye Miss American Pie.

Shannon is handling the hot house and Lyn's visit very well. Her family… Bev, Brad, and Brad’s son are set to arrive next Sunday, and we are hoping that the new A/C unit will be in place by then. Pretty shitty luck for this to happen right now. Time for bed.

May 26, 2022

It is 1:20AM, and Shannon just now came into the den and asked, “Where is Melony?” Melony is in Texas. She then asked, “Where is Mom?” Mom was long dead, of course. Shannon had a good day. We shopped for eyeglasses and ate at Chili’s. She then drove me home because I had two drinks – that’s Shannon’s limit, not mine. And she said, at some point in the day, “I’m feeling good… more PRESENT.” I agreed with her. It’s an up-and-down thing.

June 2, 2022

She has had a few good days. Brad and his son flew into Little Rock, we picked them up and drove to Jackson. Bev’s husband was not there, as he was away on business. But Shannon was able to spend three days with BOTH of her kids and one grandkid. Still, she was ready to leave a day early, and we are now back home with the broken A/C. It has been cool enough for us to survive, but Sunday is gonna be a bitch.

Stan Waters came into town and took us to dinner at Fisherman's Wharf tonight. It was GREAT to see him. He had a cool date. Ella is a mail carrier from Bossier. Stan is one of my favorite people on the planet, with street-smarts for days. Shannon did not want to go, but I shamed her into it, and she had a wonderful time. We did a little planning for the Mayo trip. That's coming up in 36 days. Fingers crossed.

June 14, 2022

This is getting more difficult every time I write. Which might explain how seldom I do. Shannon is inexorably declining. She has had some good days recently, and her mood is usually okay. Today, it was not. She awoke weepy and in generalized pain. I talked her into going for lunch, and she got a little better. Her memory is fading every day. She loses her glasses and her phone a few times every day and cannot recall names, places, and events. Still, her longer-term and more ingrained memory is good, as demonstrated by how well she does in Jeopardy. And do not even BEGIN to challenge her on rock and roll trivia.

Later today, we will go to Little Rock to see her sleep doctor, the physician who manages her C-Pap usage. Yesterday, we went to our favorite spot in the state, the Arkansas State Park at Mount Petit Jean, and the lodge/restaurant there. The lodge is incredible, with 30-foot-high wooden ceilings held up by 18-inch diameter skinned logs. It's all wood everywhere – beautifully stained in a mid-tone. Glass walls overlooking the Ozark Mountains - just breathtaking. She seemed to have a good time. I drove slowly, and she only bitched at me once.

That is some sort of record. We need to retrieve my Suzuki motorcycle from the dealer tomorrow. Lots of work has been done on it, and I need to offer it for sale. We have no other vehicle, and it appears that I may need an alternator on the Acura. I will find out tomorrow how long it will take to install. It MIGHT be a "sit and wait" job, it might require a full day. I think I really need a second car. Maybe a pickup.

June 20, 2022

We had three doctor visits this week, I went to my PCP on Tuesday... more about that later. Thursday, we saw Shannon's neurologist, Dr. Hillary Williams. She was so impressed with Shannon's condition that she almost seemed to begin to doubt her diagnosis. She had been SO convinced by Shannon's hand tremor that she jumped all over it. At the time, I thought that Shannon was exaggerating the tremor and told the Doctor. She dismissed my concern. Then. Now, not so sure.

Friday, I had the last of my back injections. The persistent pain has subsided if I am not standing. I slept in the recliner from Friday afternoon through 6AM Saturday. Shannon was very annoyed that I could not get up or even wake up. I have been depressed lately. It might be situational. I am not sure. But I resumed taking the Paxil anti-depressants, which I had not touched in five years. I told my PCP, Dr. Parish, and he asked me questions. Did I have a history of depression? Oh, for almost a decade, beginning in 2004, when my world fell apart. What is my situation? I did not tell him about certain financial threats. Still, I did tell him that taking care of Shannon has become a burden that continues to get heavier. There's no relief, and being in constant pain and gasping for breath is certainly not helping.

He then told me about HIS family. He said, and I quote as precisely as possible, "My mom had dementia for eighteen years. The last eight years, she was vegetative. My dad, a retired Air Force Lt. Colonel, sat beside her and took care of her every day. Fed her through a tube. Cleaned her up. She was his only purpose for living, and he died one month after she did." Talk about depressing. I have not stopped thinking about that conversation.

That's gonna have to do it for tonight.

Couldn't sleep, back at it. July 4th was Shannon's worst day in a while. Her tummy was upset, as it has been almost every day recently, but the real problem was her mood. She was very confused for most of the day, and I kept a close eye on her. She was also weepy, and her frustration with not understanding simple things brought her to tears. We leave for Mayo Clinic this weekend. So, getting ready for that trip is Job One. It's sort of difficult because we have no idea how long we will be gone. Two travel days up, two back, and three days scheduled for tests. I'm led to believe that there will be further tests, and more time there. Packing will be just a wild guess.

So, Shannon got a text three days ago from her friend in Natchez, one who had a liver transplant some years ago. The friend wanted to see Shannon and could come as early as this coming Saturday, and as late as the 17th. Simply the worst timing possible. Shannon asked me about it, and I said I did not favor it. We could maybe meet them for dinner on Friday, but Saturday was reserved for packing and last-minute preparations because we leave for Minnesota early Sunday. Shannon was upset. She really wanted to entertain her friend, who Shannon thought was coming to Hot Springs for a vacation. "Could we offer them our house to stay in?"

"Of course."

After sulking for a couple of hours, Shannon phoned her. It turned out that the friend would not be coming at all after realizing the inconvenience it would be for Shannon. It was not a vacation – it was a trip to see Shannon. I'm very sorry that did not work out. I want her to see friends. But right now, I gotta keep my eye on the ball. I have to get her to Minnesota and back safely, and then deal with the consequences of the trip along with my own heart issues.

July 5, 2022

I should write about a recent series of conversations with Shannon. It started with the search for a motel near Mayo. Shannon is a motel snob and cheapskate simultaneously. She will shop for hours to save $25 but wants a four-star motel. I'm not that way. I want as nice a place as we can find, very near the hospital, with a bar and room service, and I am a lousy shopper. Just give me what I want; I might not even ask for the price. Here's the deal: what I want is about fifty bucks a night more than a Motel Six. I've done this sort of thing before, and I know how much a nice hotel can improve the experience. Of all the things we have to worry about, I do not want the hotel to become an issue. Three hundred bucks or so on a trip that will cost thousands is not worth worrying about. But Shannon, who will easily spend $300 a week on LUNCH, will not let it go. So, lately we have been talking about that a lot. We have also been talking about her condition and the possibility that maybe she is not as sick as her neurologist diagnosed almost a year ago. (I do not believe that, but I often assume that she will get well. Maybe it makes her feel a little better.)

We were driving, with a pizza, to Shannon's favorite spot for a picnic and talking about that trip to the doctor. Her tremor was the subject. She said that when I first saw her tremor, I said we should "see a doctor about it immediately," and that was the first time I seemed to take her condition seriously. That's not correct, but I do understand. I've tried, rightly or wrongly, to disguise my deepest concerns.

At the neurologist's office, she was asked to hold out her right hand to display the tremor. The tremor was FAR worse than I had seen it. Her hand was vibrating - up and down RAPIDLY and maybe a couple of inches, back and forth. Based on this demonstration (after all the cognitive tests), the doctor instantly rendered her diagnosis. After a conversation, Shannon went to the restroom, and the doctor asked me a few questions. I said that I had not seen the tremor that severe, and I said that Shannon was super tense. The doctor assured me that the tremor she had witnessed was a "classic example" of a Parkinson's tremor. I told Shannon that story as we discussed whether or not the doctor had rushed to judgment. She was not happy about my answer to the doctor. "You did not believe me?"

"Of course I believed you. It's just that you were upset by the mental tests, you were totally stressed out, literally in tears, and I thought that might have contributed to the severity of the tremor." As this conversation progressed, I said, "You know you have my absolute and total support. I think you must trust me if you are to survive this. And to maintain that trust, I can never lie to you. I may not constantly voice my concerns, but, whether you like it or not, I am going to be honest with you. Bev and Brad, too. I will not hide anything or work at remembering what I said to whomever. It will be absolutely between-the-eyes the truth, every time." That smoothed things out, and we had a nice picnic.

July 5, 2022

Shannon handled the 800-mile trip well. We made Des Moines before dark on Monday, which left only 225 for today. After arriving in Rochester, Minnesota, and taking the measure of the clinic, we found a hotel directly across the street from her first appointment, Wednesday at 7:30AM. We have a suite, underground parking, a kitchen, plenty of drawers and storage, a fridge, and a microwave. The damned thing is bigger than some of my college apartments. We slept all afternoon and have a full day off tomorrow. She has early appointments on Wednesday and Thursday, so I want to find the exact spot beforehand. Shannon is sleeping comfortably now but has been quite afraid. As I have been afraid, and fearful of mentioning, a confirmation of her diagnosis by the best doctors in the world would be hope-shattering. Shannon realizes this. She cries in fear now, not just frustration, and it is heart-breaking to me. I have not changed my statements that they have it all wrong, and she will be fine. It is a telling thing when we are hoping for something as insidious as Parkinson's Disease. She is seeing more hallucinations now and awoke with one last night at the Des Moines hotel. I'll try to keep you guys informed as this adventure continues.

July 13, 2022

Today, we got the worst news possible from the smartest doctors in the world. Shannon's diagnosis was confirmed. We were told that our only course is to manage her medications and keep her as safe as possible. Particularly locks on the outside doors to prevent her from sleepwalking into the great outdoors.

The most enlightening and frankly scary thing we learned was this: the only way to predict her future decline rate is to examine the rate of past decline. If we want to know how far she might decline in the coming year, then examine the decline since last year and project that same amount of decline into next year. THAT is some difficult stuff. How many "weepy days" did she have last year? How many days of depression, how much time in bed, how many hallucinations, how many episodes of sleepwalking? Keeping a journal is SO unlike me. I have never done it before. Upon hearing this, I realized why I felt compelled to keep it. I suppose that it is the best I can do, but there won't be tally sheets. Just all by feel, I guess. Shannon took the news in stride. I think she left the denial and bargaining phases some time ago and is now resigned. Acceptance is to come. Right?

I should write a few words about the Mayo Clinic. It is both extravagant and unassuming at the same time. Both opulent and homey. Hard to describe. The employees are extraordinary! All are polite, helpful, and as professional as a pro baseball umpire. The physicians wear suits and ties and polished dress shoes. No lab coats here. Shannon's PCP in Little Rock works in sweatpants… he would be a janitor at Mayo. When they sit with you, they listen carefully, often repeating what you said or nodding in understanding. When they speak, it is in measured language and tone, with authority. They speak in a way that builds trust and confidence, even when the news is as bad as today's.

We walked from the hospital through downtown Rochester to a wonderful Italian restaurant, overate, and then slept all afternoon. We awoke at 8PM, and pondered options. Shannon has one more scan tomorrow at 7:30AM, and a final consultation at 3:30PM. We'll stay here Thursday night and depart Friday.

July 19, 2022

We left Minnesota Friday afternoon, and spent the night in Cedar Rapids, Iowa. We spent the next night in St. Louis and had a great Italian dinner with my son, Dave and his girlfriend, Erin. Dave even picked up the check. He's leaving in a few days for a couple of weeks in Italy, base jumping off cliffs. We arrived home before sundown on Sunday and slept until Monday night. Both of us were totally exhausted. Now, Tuesday night, we are returning to normal.

Shannon has been in sad shape since we got home. She's weepy and depressed and finding new ailments daily. Yesterday, it was her big toe. Today, that has spread to the leg. We are facing a potentially back-breaking financial issue. Travis Hargrave is threatening to withhold my monthly payments of $4,000. We can make it without his payments, but it will be tight. I talked with Shannon about it. About ways to cut expenses. Less dining out. Less gasoline. We will be cutting back on A/C use, cable TV, and several life insurance policies. And I am gonna sue Travis. I have about $15,000 that I can dedicate to that, and more in credit if necessary. I am not gonna lose. Being unable to take Shannon to lunch every day is a problem. It's one of the few ways that I can get her to leave the house. Damn, managing this is difficult. Shannon's short-term memory is almost non-existent. She becomes upset about the smallest things and obsesses over others. The more manic she becomes, the kinder I react. That's not my first impulse, but it IS how I respond.

"From: Bev

Sent: Tuesday, July 19, 2022 4:50 PM

To: David

Cc: Brad; Macy

Subject: Re: today's journal

Thank you for the update. Would you mind sharing the details of what the doctor said, is there a treatment plan of sorts? Will she see these docs again? Will they be directly involved in her treatment? Any changes made to her treatment etc.

Many thanks!

Bev"

My response.

"Bev,

It actually appeared to me that the doctor's mind was about 50% made up before meeting us. He had the Arkansas notes. He performed many of the same physical tests that were done in Arkansas. I'm talking about dexterity, reflex, orientation, walking.

And a few of the mental tests… not nearly as many, and Shannon blew off the four-hour mental marathon test that had upset her so much in Little Rock. He recommended a slight increase in her dosage of Exelon, agreed completely with Hillary on everything else, and said that Hillary "was right on top of this." He only continued with the brain MRI because it was pre-approved by insurance. He had the results for our final consultation and showed us a series of brain images. The color images clearly displayed abnormal areas, though they were not strikingly abnormal… blue instead of red.

He will not be involved in the future, unless we ask for his help. He advised us to accelerate the items on our bucket list (what he actually said, word for word, is burned into my memory – "If you have a 'bucket list', now is the time to empty it") travel soon instead of waiting, get lots of exercise and sunshine, work crossword puzzles… in short, remain as active as possible. I am trying, but it is getting more difficult daily.

David"

July 23, 2022

As a real estate broker, one of my favorite associates was Jan Rudnick. She is a caretaker for her husband Ron, who is very ill. (Note: Jan and I have compared notes for years, and Ron died before Shannon.)

Instant Message to Jan Rudnick in Long Island, NY

"Jan, I have come to a strategy. Remember how I used to teach 'if someone cuts you off in traffic, instead of getting pissed, do something nice for the next guy. Don't be a mirror and reflect bad vibes, be a pillow and absorb them.'"

So, as her illness progresses, she becomes more forgetful, hallucinatory, and frankly meaner. At first, I became more frustrated and angry. But, after thinking it through, I decided to become ever kinder, ever more gentle, ever more patient. It is sometimes difficult, but I'm getting better. And it's helping me even if it doesn't help her. The difficulty in dealing with a mental issue is that their behavior OFTEN SEEMS SO OUTRAGEOUS THAT IT MUST BE FAKE. But it is no more fake than a heart attack. This is not something that you can simply learn, it must be inculcated into your mental process. That takes time and patience. Not just with her, but with myself, too. I AM getting better, but I honestly dread years of it."

July 28, 2022

Last weekend, Steve, Shannon's nephew, was planning to come visit Shannon, and I kept it a secret from her, as a surprise. But he had issues with his eyes and only made it halfway. So, he called me, and we packed up and went to help him in Noname, Texas. We had dinner, talked, and he and Shannon looked through a box of photos he brought along. Then, before he left our motel room to go to his, he and Shannon hugged for what seemed like five minutes. They just stood still, holding one another. It was poignant. Jenni, Shannon's niece, came to the motel with her husband the next morning, and we convinced Steve to allow them to escort him home. Good thing, too. He only made it thirty minutes before his eyes failed him. We drove home.

Digression

Steve is a real piece of work. A user of, ah, questionable substances for many years, he was always loaded with money. While we were traveling, Shannon borrowed ten thousand dollars from him. She paid on it faithfully until it was down to three thousand, at which time

Steve said to Shannon, "That's enough, don't pay me anymore. I have plenty, do not worry about the rest." So, Shannon stopped repaying. I was not worried about it, just slightly bothered.

The last time Steve visited us, he was down on his luck. He had lost his source of income. I asked Steve to walk out onto our deck with me, for privacy. There I said, "Steve, I think we still owe you about three thousand dollars, is that right?"

"Yes," he said.

"I want to pay you back, here in the next few days. Is that OK?

Steve did not hesitate. "I could really use it right now."

I had ten one-hundred-dollar bills folded into my pocket and gave them to him. "Two thousand more when the banks open."

My son Dave is in Italy, wingsuit jumping off cliffs. His live-in girlfriend has gone nuts. She authored a blast of Facebook posts that remind me so much of my own late sister, who began a lifelong bi-polar battle at age twenty-two, same as her. I contacted Dave through FB Messenger (his iPhone would not text or call from Italy), and he was concerned about a .22 rifle and certain other items that he would rather she and the police not see. Her actions could easily prompt the police to visit the apartment. I messaged Dave about this at 4PM today, and by 6PM, Shannon and I were on the road to his St. Louis apartment. We drove into Missouri, about 125 miles from Dave's apartment, before stopping for the night. Hopefully, the manager will let us into his apartment tomorrow. We intend to swoop in, clean the place of questionable items, and then haul ass back home.

Shannon is having a hard time. She is sleeping, but she awoke a moment ago to ask, "Where is Debbie?"

"There's no Debbie here," I told her. She has had a number of these hallucinations recently. It is definitely getting worse. Last night, I awoke at 3AM and needed to pee. I heard her calling me weakly from her room. She could not get out of bed because her good knee was locked up and hurting. So, now we are shopping for a walkie-talkie and three foolproof door locks.

July 30, 2022

Shannon did great on the rest of the trip. No pain or complaints. A little bossy about some of the details, but I had it thought out, and it worked like a charm. The apartment manager could not be found, but we did find a locksmith, got inside, and scooped up the stuff. We then met the next-door neighbor, a harmless 80-year-old man, and gave him one of the new keys. And hauled ass. Back home, after 850 miles, before dark. Twenty-three hours. Amazing.

Later, David would say, "I was so worried about her that I was not jumping, just hanging out at the hotel, watching my vacation collapse. Then, when I knew you were on it, I relaxed and had a good time." That made me feel like a dad, again.

Today and tonight, Shannon has had it rough. She thought that she had left a couple of smoker's pipes on the dining table and freaked out. I told her it was ok… no big deal. But she started whimpering about how she "cannot do anything right." I told her that I did not want to hear it. Waypoint is a tiny casual lakeside spot in Hot Springs Village, and we were stopping there for a sandwich. Once there, she began to whine about needing a therapist. I asked why. She said that no one would listen to her. "Bev shut me out… you shut me out…" I argued that I hadn't, and she said, "See, you just did." And she was right, I had. Damn, I am trying to be better about that stuff, but I still fail.

Tonight, she came into the den crying. She said that she really wants to go to Arizona to be with her family in August. This is a full family reunion, and her ex, Danny, will be there with Bev and Brad. Liz told her, on the phone, "Mom, I don't want you to come if you can't handle it. I can't take care of you." I told her that I would take her to Arizona. Heart, lungs, altitude, and all… I'll take you. I am so disappointed in her kids that I could spit. I told Shannon how I felt, and she asked, "Why?" I replied, "What would you give to spend an hour with your dad?"

Sometime in the next 48 hours, I am gonna talk to Brad. I can't talk to Bev. Whatever I say angers her, and goes straight to Shannon.

August 7, 2022

I did not talk to Brad… I'm almost afraid to… afraid that I'd tell him what I REALLY think. He texted Shannon and Bev, saying I was NOT on the list and that it would be awkward if I was there. So, Shannon called it off. Then, after chewing on it for a couple of days, I thought, "I can simply take Shannon there for the Saturday party while I hide for the day and evening at a bar in Sedona." She called her ex-husband Dan, and he was all for it. That sounded good to Shannon… then bad… then good… then bad. So, I don't know what is gonna happen, but I did tell Shannon, "It is almost always a mistake to pass on something that might only happen once." Many times, I have put something off, only to discover that it could never happen again. Would any of us have missed the LAST Beatles concert, if we had known it was the last? But there always IS a last. I fear that for Shannon, this is the last chance to see her original nuclear family, at least before her decline into dementia. The idea that I would somehow resent her former husband, and cause awkwardness, is preposterous. I feel as if I am fighting a losing battle, just like Shannon.

August 12, 2022

Lots to write about tonight.

First, we are not in Arizona. After I worked out a plan to go, one which kept me completely out of the get together, Bev sent a note to Shannon, and she decided not to go. Shannon felt like she would be unwelcome there. Brad did not answer my message at all. I am so disappointed in those two that it is all I can do to stay out of it. Shannon was in tears, and I was just angry. We went through several on/off stages of this.

Bev and Brad have both told me, "We are here for you… anything you need, anytime… we want to help." I came very close to sending them a text: "Remember when you guys promised to help me with Shannon? Well, you are off the hook… you can stop now… you have helped enough." Tonight, Shannon said that Bev wants to spend a weekend with her in Memphis this September. Was that OK with me? Of course, it is. Why would it not be? Well, you will have to take me over there and come get me. No problem, I said. I would take you anywhere to see your son or daughter. As Roy Orbison sang with the Traveling Wilburys, "Anything you need, you got it." Bev is trying to make up for the Arizona thing, even Shannon can see that.

My heart/breathing/weight issues are getting better. I've lost 25 pounds… just 40 to go. When I switched physicians after A YEAR at Christus, I could not walk to the mailbox without getting winded. Now, I am walking a couple of miles in the streets and doing a few weights, too. The back is better but not perfect, but my left leg is hurting a lot. I might need another injection.

August 13, 2022

Groundhog Day.

Every damned day is exactly like the last one. I wake up, and Cricket is sleeping at the foot of the bed. As I sit up, she does, as well, and I say, "Morning girl," as she yawns and stretches. I move toward the bathroom as she eyes me to determine if I am gone for good or coming right back. Once she decides that I am up for the day, she stands beside her food bowl. I take pills. If my back hurts, I add a couple of ibuprofen. I grab a bottle of water and a peach on my way to the recliner. I will spend most of the day there. Shannon will shuffle down the hall, stop to ask if I am ok, and grab a protein bar before going back to her bedroom, where she will spend most of the rest of the day. At some point, she will come back and ask if we can go to Sonic or Waypoint for a sandwich. (If I make a turkey and tomato sandwich on whole grain toast, it does not pass her test for food. If it is not mass-produced and wrapped in foil, it's not food.) This will invariably happen at three or four o'clock, just in time to ruin her appetite for dinner. I probably have a filet mignon, salmon, or fresh chicken set out, but now I have to cook it for myself. Which I probably will not do.

After walking the street for an hour, I'll retreat to my recliner, have another bottle of water… just one Coke a day… and watch TV until I might sleep between midnight and 5:00 AM. Most nights, I sleep in the recliner to be nearby in case Shannon sleepwalks. She will show up in the den, wondering through a sleep-haze where her daughter or son or, most recently, cousin Debby are sleeping tonight. Basement? Bedroom? "No, baby… you've been dreaming." And I escort her back to bed, probably lying with her until she is again asleep. Then I can go to my own bed, arrange the pillows just so, putting as little pressure on my troubled rotator cuffs as possible, and drift off. That's my day. That's her day. At least once weekly, we go to Little Rock or

Hot Springs to see doctors, and there is at least one Walgreens stop every week. On Sundays, we sit on her bed and sort pills into three seven-pocket dividers. A large one for morning pills, a medium size for lunch time, and a small for those three of four that she takes at bedtime. That's my groundhog week.

Tonight, I got a message from Jeff. He and Izzy are driving home to California from Maine in their motorhome and may stop in to see us on October 7th. (How in the hell he could know, seven weeks in advance, where he will be on October 7th is beyond my limited understanding.) When we last visited them on their trawler in 2015, I said something (exactly what I do not remember) that implied that Shannon was not smart. He repeated something about that conversation in an email, and Shannon read it. Now she thinks that Jeff is an asshole, when it was my statement. I may have to tell Jeff not to come. Not a tragedy, but it is another something to deal with.

While in the car on the way to see Lyn and Judy Cathey, Shannon talked to Bev. They talked for at least fifteen minutes… me listening to Shannon's side the entire time. I guess I am not gonna get over the Tiger Stadium incident and the fact that Shannon is not in Arizona right now.

August 31, 2022

Jenni, Trey, and Steve are coming to visit this weekend. Apparently, they intend to stay only one night. Next week, we are going on a trip. We hope to spend the first night in Chattanooga, then on to see Charlie and Kathy in Virginia Beach for a couple of days of guitar playing. Oh, I need that. Then, hopefully, we can travel up the east coast as far as New England. I also need lobster!

Shannon is freaked out about the whole thing. Wants a new car before we leave. That's gonna be hard, but at least it is possible because

Travis has paid me for August. We filed suit against him for non-payment just last Friday; he got the papers on the 23rd. And the check was dated August 18, postmarked on the 26th, and received on the 30th. So, it looks like the check was written last week and left on the desk until the papers were served, then mailed the next business day. If this is the end of it, then I feel good about it. If he tries to delay payment again, I do not know what to do except proceed with the suit.

Shannon's confusion and frankly thoughtless behavior toward me has really intensified. She freaks out whenever we are expecting company, so tomorrow, I must clean and mow despite being scarcely able to walk. The back thing is killing me and hurts all the time. Another injection is scheduled for 8:30AM Friday.

September 7, 2022 - 2AM

We left home yesterday at 12:47PM and drove 400 miles to Nashville, arriving at 9PM and eating Wendy's on the bed.

Shannon was a real trooper. No complaining, lots of help. She IS dingy. Terrible short-term memory. But compliant. We hope to attend a Van Gogh exhibit tomorrow before leaving. We'll drive deep into the night, rest up, and drive the rest of the way to Virginia Beach on Thursday. We will get a motel there for Thursday and Friday night. Charlie and I will chill on Friday, then Saturday sailing, and Sunday...Willie Nelson!

Monday, we leave for New York City and, hopefully a Broadway show. Then, Vermont and maybe Niagara Falls. The doctors at Mayo said we should empty the bucket list, and we are trying.

Shannon told me that she awoke yesterday morning and was unable to recall the year, 2022. She was confused. She thought Patti died in 2022, so this MUST be 2024. She is constantly confused and frustrated by dates. And numbers. Appointments, of which she has many, sometimes leave her in a tearful panic.

We packed two weeks of drugs... two packages of three containers each. Morning, noon, and evening pills. Next week's pills are banded together. So, tonight she, in confusion, opened that pack. If there is one thing I have to do, it's keep that stuff straight, so I got on her pretty hard. We decided that I'll keep the pills. More and more, it's falling on me.

Thankfully, our financial situation is improving. We filed suit against Hargrave, and he paid up instantly. Shannon is now, for the first time ever, contributing by paying $190 a month to the HOA for dues and water, which still leaves her with a grand a month and no other bills. With no mortgage payment now, the total freed up to me is about $1500 monthly. That's real money. I can set aside about an extra fifteen thousand a year in cash. Mattress money for the day that she needs 24/7 care. Gimme three years, and we might be able to keep her comfortable. That is now my only goal. If I can keep her out of the corral at a nursing home, her greatest fear, I'll feel successful.

Jenni and Trey came to visit last weekend. Jenni is very kind, and Trey is interesting. Still, it was exhausting, and we both slept eighteen of the next twenty-four hours after they departed. Here's the deal: people want to see Shannon now, before (they presume) she fades too far. They do not realize the strain those visits put on Shannon. She cleans for days, and worries her ass off, often crying real tears of frustration and back pain. Then, I get the job of buying groceries, cooking every-damned-thing, entertaining, planning, and cleaning. The visitors mean well, and I want Shannon to get a lot of this, but something has to give. Housekeepers and caterers, maybe. We'll figure it out. This got very real, very quickly.

September 9, 2022

Two days in Virginia Beach, now. Dinner tonight with Charlie and Kathy. Tomorrow, we are going sailing on Charlie's catamaran, Festival. Shannon is getting a lot of sleep and rest yet remains very tired. So, sailing and dinner tomorrow, stay with Charlie and Kathy tomorrow and Sunday night. Then, maybe, head north. I don't think Shannon wants to extend this trip. So, we might go straight home.

There was an unusual event tonight. Shannon was trying to reach Brad, by text. I'm not sure which buttons she pressed, but suddenly, there were numerous notifications on her phone from other folks, and Shannon took that to mean that Brad had been injured. She was panic-stricken. I held her closely, read her phone, and said, "Shannon, I am not sure what caused this on your phone, but I am CERTAIN that Brad is just fine." She calmed down, and Brad was fine.

September 14, 2022

We are home. Shannon was very tired and insisted we come directly home from Virginia Beach. We spent the first night in Hickory, NC, then drove over 700 miles Tuesday to get home at about 10PM. Shannon did very well on the trip. That's a LONG drive for anyone, but she held up… once she finally decided to. About five hours from home, near Jackson, TN, she began calling hotels. I asked, "Do you want to stop?" And she would say "no" but then continue to call more hotels. Then, we hit Taco Bell, and thus satiated she hunkered down, and we finished the drive.

September 19, 2022

Today was Shannon's worst day yet, specifically in reference to hallucinations. Throughout the day, she "heard" knocking and scratching sounds from inside her bedroom and outside the windows. She called me into the bedroom several times. “Did you hear that?” “Oh, c’mon, you MUST have heard that!” The sounds she described seemed to me like those that a mouse might make. She even said so as she looked under the bed for the noisemakers. I believe that her rat phobia had something to do with it.

Then tonight, after retiring to bed, she came into the den and asked me, “Where is that black kid that was standing at my bed?” She was partially dreaming, but frightened. I went to bed with her, and she fell asleep. But it was a fitful sleep, and she cried out several times in just an hour or so. I made an excuse, saying that I was going to make a sandwich, so that I could have a few minutes to write this. While in the kitchen, making my sandwich, she came in.

“I thought you were going out to get a sandwich. Then I thought, “Where can he get a sandwich at this hour?” Today, she wanted to go to Lowe’s… then she didn’t… then she did… then Walmart… then… you get the picture.

September 20, 2022

OK, so here is the latest on the hallucinations. Three days ago, we left messages for Hillary to call us. We remembered that she had offered to prescribe something for hallucinations, if we ever needed it. We left a message on the hospital’s portal. After leaving the message, Shannon asked me every couple of hours if there was an answer. There wasn’t. Shannon was in tears. Really frustrated and afraid of these noises. The next day, Friday, we left another message, and the nurse practitioner called us back at 3pm. She said the problem could be a urinary tract infection, and she would only prescribe the drug Seroquel if Shannon was tested for that first. We dashed to the doc-in-a-box and had the test, which was, of course, negative. The drug was prescribed. Shannon texted Bev and Brad to tell them. Both thought she should not take the drug. There was a flurry of texts back and forth, I became annoyed, Shannon stressed out, and we picked up the drug. Then Shannon decided not to take it UNLESS the sounds got worse. Of course, the sounds went away. What a cluster. Shannon is getting worse every day. Today, she said, "I was so good for a year, and now I am falling apart." Well, she WASN'T good for the last year. She IS worse now, but the fade has been happening for at least two years. Only now is it so apparent. She has great trouble finding words, stays in bed all day, weeps a lot, slumps around the house in pajamas, and hasn't smiled in days. It is hard to watch, and hard to be around. It's just hard.

October 3, 2022

We have entered a terrible stage. As we departed Jackson, after a short visit there, Shannon began to cry and cried for hours. While sleeping together in a double bed in Jackson, Shannon had several episodes – while sleeping- on both nights. She would begin to groan and thrash, increasing in intensity until she screamed out loud. Sometimes, it's not a full scream, more of a cry. Each time, I nudged her gently and calmed her with a few words. In the morning, she would not remember. I think Bev finally gets it. She watched her mom all weekend and then texted us on the way home. She wants to come visit us early next month, after not visiting Shannon for several months.

Then today, the shit really hit the fan. Shannon's aural hallucinations worsened..."like a ceiling fan in my head," and she took a pill to sleep. When she awoke this afternoon and came into the den, she thought her mother had given her the pill, and that I was her dad. Most scary is the fact that it took several minutes for her to regain her grip. She called for her mom. She asked where she was and asked several times if I was her dad. Tonight, her behavior has been very erratic and almost robotic.

She began to talk again about suicide. Nothing playful about it this time. All of the firearms are unloaded, and the ammunition is hidden. She wouldn't know how to either load or fire any of them, but I am taking no chances. Damn.

October 7, 2022

We have clearly entered an entirely new stage in Shannon's illness. She is constantly confused. I mean well over half the time. The confusion leads to frustration, then to tears of anger and impotence. I do not understand the disease, but I understand this. Today, we went to see a new doctor in Little Rock. He's a good guy, a good listener, and ready to take action. He insisted that Shannon take the Seroquel. He says it will quiet her night terrors. Several months ago, I wrote a song," You Can Have What's Left of Me" bemoaning her mental descent and my matching physical decline. First verse:

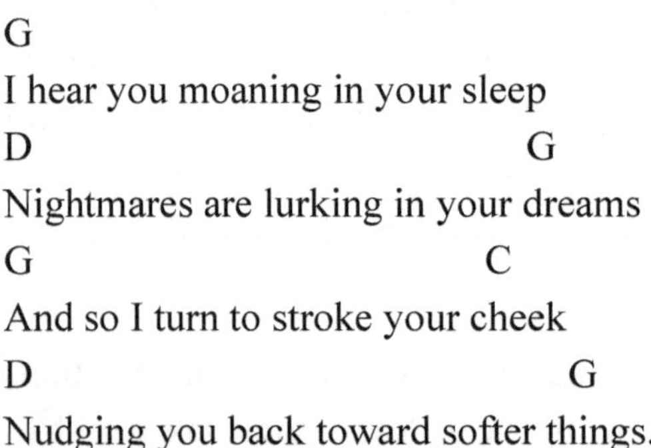
```
G
I hear you moaning in your sleep
D                                  G
Nightmares are lurking in your dreams
G                              C
And so I turn to stroke your cheek
D                                    G
Nudging you back toward softer things.
```

She is now crying out several times a night, her LBD-afflicted mind searching for peace or racing away from dragons. Who knows? But today, after a trip to Little Rock and a stop at Chili's, she freaked out as she tried to re-assemble her CPAP mask. She will not listen to me. I try to gently show her the steps, and that fails. I try harder, more emphatically- no luck. Finally, instead of losing patience I do it myself. I am really trying. Really.

October 16, 2022

Wrote this to Bev tonight:

> "Shannon fell again today. I heard her calling for me from my bedroom. She had tripped on her heater cord and was flat on her back, sort of awkwardly squeezed by a chair. She wanted to go to the doc-in-a-box, and we did, but they were busy. Shannon was impatient, so we went home. I think she was more frightened than hurt, and she hasn't complained this evening. I have had broken ribs three times. And they hurt like hell. If you sneeze or laugh, you feel excruciating pain. And it does not get better quickly… two or three weeks to see any improvement and six weeks all in. I do not think she broke anything, but stretching that cartilage is just as painful."
>
> Dave"

The real issue is, "How am I gonna watch her?" I can stop her from going outside unsupervised, but damn, this happened in her bedroom. I really need a communication system. Something like a baby monitor, but not continuous. It needs to be set off by a yell or a crash - not the normal sounds of sleep.

Her mental state has been better today, ribs and all. The list of things that confuse her and that she cannot remember, dates, appointments, what day of the week is today… all of that is worsening rapidly. She says, "I cannot understand how I went for a year without any real symptoms, then suddenly I am seeing things and thinking you are my mother. What the hell is going on?" She is asking, "Why me?" a lot.

"What did I do to get this?" Those questions just slay me. There are no answers, of course, but that is no help.

October 29, 2022

This was a pretty good week, all in all. We arose very early Tuesday morning to attend a trial hearing in Bossier City – part of the lawsuit against Travis. Shannon was reluctant to drive down, attend the hearing, and return in a single day. But she falls often, and I cannot leave her at home. She presented several ideas for staying home or making the trip easier. So, on Sunday, when she came to me with another implausible idea, I said, "Shannon, I need you. I need you to be as strong as possible and help me with this. To help US with this."

Her reaction was amazing. She stiffened, brightened, and said, "OK, whatever you need." And she did it. God, I love her. We awoke at 5AM and drove to Bossier City. Upon arriving home at 4PM, we both slept for 18 hours.

Friday, we had to do it again. This time, it was a spinal epidural injection for me. Gotta be over a dozen by now. We awoke at 4:30AM to be at the surgical center by 6:30. Shannon never complained. Then, she drove home as I was still partially sedated. I'm afraid to let her out on her own, but she did well. And again, we slept for hours.

She is very confused by upcoming events. This is happening in the next few weeks.

1. On Monday, We are driving to Memphis to see my son David. The housekeeper is scheduled for the same day. I have it worked out, but Shannon is upset.

2. Bev is coming to visit on the following Friday, November 4th. LSU plays on Saturday, and Bev returns to Jackson on Sunday. Shannon is apoplectic about that.

3. Thanksgiving is in late November, and we are going to Jackson. My son David is moving from St. Louis to Southern California. These two overlapping events have Shannon in a tizzy. I answered at least fifty questions yesterday and today about those dates. Oh, and it is complicated by several doctor visits. I am a walking calendar.

She has become incredibly finicky about her diet. I just want her to eat healthily. But a Sonic burger and Lean Cuisine is all that she will eat. Well, that and pizza. I just KNOW that a few veggies and some real nutrition are necessary, and frankly, eating dinner is one of the few things we can do together. Tonight, turning up her nose at a filet mignon, she declared,

"I just don't want meat anymore."

"Hamburgers?" I asked

"Well, those are covered with stuff."

"Ooookaaaay." Tomorrow is another day.

November 3, 2022

How appropriate. Today, I woke, bright and alert, at ten AM. I turned on the TV, and a rerun of Groundhog Day was on. It was one of my all-time favorite movies until I began living it. Every day is like the last. Oh, the doctors and the trips to Little Rock are a little different, but not really. Yesterday we went to Little Rock for a scheduled appointment with an internist. They wanted to do a colonoscopy on Shannon. I think it's just a new doctor trying to generate revenue. But no way! Can you imagine? You have a patient with a terminal brain disease, and you want to stick a probe up her butt? And one more thing. She was being visited by a couple of interns who were asking her questions and trying to learn something from her ailment. At some point Shannon mentioned that she might sometimes wake in the evening and drink a Diet Coke. Now, I will not take the reader on a digression into Diet Coke, though I easily could. Suffice it to say that she drinks several a day and has for years. I tried to get her to taper off years ago, but she wouldn't. Now, what does it matter? She LIKES them, and that's enough for me. So, upon hearing the words "Diet Coke", these two young men were on her like a cougar on a duck. "You can't do that…the caffein…your sleep…"

I said, "Hold on there, fellas. Shannon has a terminal illness. No one is going to tell her that she cannot have a Coke." I sometimes feel like I am in a novel by Kafka. Nothing makes sense, but everything does.

At about 11PM last night, Shannon came into the den. "I just woke up and called Bev to ask her where she is." Of course, Bev is in Jackson. But, according to Shannon, Bev did not protest the call. She is beginning to understand.

Shannon wants to go to Arizona at Christmas. I'll get her a plane ticket, but I'm not going. We shall see. She has lots of time to change her mind between now and then.

November 8, 2022

Email to Charlie, Vince, Kent, and my kids.

> "I spoke with my attorney about the lawsuit last week. (I've paid about twenty and have about 25 more before the soup gets thin.) He said that might not be enough. So, Sunday night, I put the 1973 D18 and the 0015M (Martin guitars) for sale on Reverb. com. D18 brought 2K. The 0015, $1250. Both are gone, less than 48 hours from ad to ship. So that's both motorcycles and two fine Martin guitars dedicated now to this fight. That D-18 was 6 months old when I bought it from Duane King. It went from "new" to "vintage" while

> hanging on my walls. As Emmy Lou sang, "I've grown used to losing what I'm fondest of."
>
> Dave"

Shannon continues her dive into the clouds. Last week, she thought I was her mother, and it took me five minutes to convince her otherwise. That adds a bit of importance to the lawsuit, although I have to say I am ready for a fight.

November 18, 2022

I gotta say, I am really struggling now. I'm more patient and kinder to Shannon than ever. Mostly because I've grown accustomed to her lapses, and I have accepted that she cannot help it. But the inability to keep dates in her mind is so frustrating. "When are we going to Jackson?" she asks. "Wednesday the 23rd," I answer. Over and over, maybe five or six times a day.

We have two trips coming up. One to Jackson for Thanksgiving and the other to DFW airport where Shannon will board a non-stop flight to Phoenix. Brad will pick her up and take her to his home in Arizona. I'm worried about getting her to the gate. She'll be gone from December 20 through 26. I intend to hang around Texas and visit old friends and my 90-year-old cousin, JoAnn. In addition to that, Bev, her husband, and son Brian are coming HERE on December 16th for the weekend. Jeez, that is a lot of sugar for a dime. I'll start the new year like the last sixty or so - exhausted.

November 27, 2022

We are back from the Jackson Thanksgiving, and the story is too long to cover right now. There is one step in Shannon's decline that I want to document tonight. She has become much more belligerent. She is far more easily insulted. I am not going to write them all down, but every day for the last five days, she has found something to get angry about. It always is baseless, and she always gets over it quickly. But it IS a change, and I fear it will worsen. We are going to see the Eagles tonight in Little Rock. I have given up drinking and most meats. "Losing weight without speed eating sunflower seeds, drinking lots of carrot juice, and soaking up rays." Cheeseburger in Paradise, Jimmy Buffet.

December 14, 2022

I've been negligent and not keeping up as I should. Shannon has created a monster with the pre-Christmas get-together. It looks as if we may have as many as eight visitors on Saturday. Thankfully, I can walk again after a painful bout with gout over the last three days. We bought a pre-fab Christmas dinner for Saturday, and Bev's husband is set to cook gumbo on Sunday. Bev has Covid and expects to be non-contagious by their Saturday arrival. Shannon, again, has worked herself into a frenzy. I PROMISE that I will not allow this to happen again. It's just too much for her. The problem is, of course, that Shannon truly wants and needs to see her nieces, nephews, son and daughter, and Bryan, the step-grandson whom she cherishes. They want and need to see her, as well. There'll come a time when she will not recognize them. As my LBD reading predicts, her annoyance, frustration, and belligerence factors are ramping up. One can spend an hour with her and think she is just fine. We still laugh, joke, play music trivia, and have good times together, but we spend more and more time in tense and stressful situations. I've adjusted well to that, though. If she wants something done, I either do it or gently explain why I cannot. Darn, I'm driving slower, talking less profanely, and being gentler with everyone. Go figure.

Shannon's short-term memory continues to worsen. If you spend a day with her, she will ask for help about twenty times. Today, she forgot twice how to work her TV remote and had three "problems" with her phone. And she has zero confidence - asking me if it is okay to throw away a wrinkled tomato, for example. Today, I needed $85 for the housekeeper, and I had only twenty-dollar bills. I asked Shannon if she had five bucks, and she came back with two singles, thinking that was what I needed. Tonight, she asked me four times in thirty minutes when she was leaving for Phoenix, argued with me twice about it, and finally said, "Well, you handle it." Of course, that is what I've done. It's what I am doing. All the way down to meeting a friend at DFW airport who will guard the car while I negotiate a way to get her successfully to the gate. The weekly housekeeper has been a blessing. Expensive, but worth it. I may have written previously that I intend to increase the frequency gradually as Shannon's needs increase. Ultimately, I will switch to a caregiver/housekeeper before reaching the 24/7 point. I do not have a plan for that. Of course, this depends on winning the lawsuit in Bossier City. There has been a slow period lately, so there have been no recent charges. But it is already up to about twenty grand, and I have another five on retainer with the attorney and add to it monthly. This would not have been possible without the mortgage trick last April. As God is my witness, I am gonna win this thing. I'd sure better, because I have bet the farm on it.

December 19, 2022

Well, Arizona is a no-go. Shannon is afraid to travel, and I think that's a good thing. The pre-Christmas weekend went off without a hitch. Holly and her three kids were here, as were Bev, her husband, and Brian. Complete with two dogs and two cats, there were fifteen souls in this little home. Everyone got fed, everyone got presents, and everyone got home safely.

Bev is furious with me. She wrote a lengthy email that basically called me disrespectful for repeating the things she said to her mom. Here is my journal entry, which was emailed to Bev and Brad, Bev's reply emails to me, and my follow-up. (Get ready…cover your ears.)

My journal entry, emailed to Bev and Brad.

> "Lately, Shannon has been really upset… I mean to the point of crying for a couple of days… about a conversation she had with Bev while in Jackson. Shannon thinks I am likely to die before her, and she says Bev told her, "I won't take you in." I get that, of course. Bev has a family of her own. But it knocked Shannon on her ass. Shannon has told me for years that she had Bev to rely on, but now says she must have misunderstood and that Bev does not intend to house her in her final stage. Actually, Bev does not intend to house her at all. Her final stage will almost certainly be a memory care/nursing home environment. And if I can keep my aching heart beating till then, she'll be here until that happens. In for a penny, in for a pound."

Bev, very angry, responded on Dec 15, 2022 at 7:29 PM.

> "I must say this email is pretty upsetting and unfair towards me. It feels inflammatory and directed at me. Such a delicate topic needs to be addressed directly. I will not discuss this with you over email. I will also not discuss it without Brad involved. Meaning, that I will not talk about it with you face-to-face this weekend unless we conference Brad in.
>
> Bev"

From: Bev

Sent**:** Saturday, December 17, 2022 7:46 AM

To: David, Brad

Subject: Re: Tonight's journal entry

"Good morning,

It seems there is a lot of confusion right now and a lack of effective communication between all of us. This is no doubt an incredibly stressful, frightening, and disorienting time for all of us for similar and for different reasons. We each have our own unique experience of grief and fear. Communication between families is hard as it is, particularly during times of crisis. This is exacerbated by the fact that we only became a "family" later in our lives - we don't have much history together, nor have we been able to build deeper relationships together as a cohesive family. There is nothing inherently wrong with that, it is normal and natural when folks remarry later in life. It does create less of a foundation and bond from which to work together in a time of crisis, though. Furthermore, we each likely have our own ideas about what is "best" for mom. It is my belief that what is "best" for mom right now is that we find a way to communicate effectively and respectfully, and some ground rules need to be laid to facilitate that communication.

I think that Brad's proposal to come out here is a good one. At a minimum, if he doesn't come out here in person, we at least need to have a very serious and candid discussion about the trajectory of mom's illness - from a practical standpoint regarding the various options for her care and living situation. It is my understanding that mom is confused and scared about what will happen should she outlive David. This is a difficult topic, I don't want to talk about David's mortality, and I'm sure he doesn't either. Moreover, we cannot predict the future. She is scared though, so allaying her fears and making sure she has a clear sense of what her circumstances might be seems important. She deserves to feel a sense of security and safety - she is anxious enough as it is. Whatever we can do to ease her fears seems like the loving thing.

I will not be able to house her if and when she needs 24/7 care. David, you have said you cannot do that either if she ends up needing 24/7 care. I am reserving my feelings about the things you suggested in your email here, albeit difficult not to defend myself. The objective truth is that it will not be tenable for her to live in my home if, at any point, she cannot live with David and needs round-the-clock care. I have thought long, hard, and painstakingly about this and have very serious and real reasons for this decision, and I request that everyone respect that. To imply that I am not reliable or that I am selfish is cruel and does not take into account my subjectivity or my deeply personal reasons for this.

As aforementioned, it is my understanding that David, you are not going to be able to keep her in your home if she needs 24/7 care and I assume the same is true for Brad and Stacy. (Again please correct me if wrong.) I do not judge either of you for that. I respect your reasons and trust your judgment. Whatever the case, it is imperative that we talk about what the various possible scenarios are and what the plan will be in those scenarios.

I would like to propose that we keep all communication very respectful moving forward. I realize that we are all hurting and feeling pain and need support. Respectfully, I would prefer not to receive any more emails like the one you sent David. I would also prefer not to receive anymore journal entries in general and prefer that communication be more direct and respectful overall.

With love,

Bev"

THAT is a lot of word salad, but it basically says that Bev is unwilling to invest her time in caring for her mother.

I did not see either email until tonight, the 19th. This was my answer to both:

"Well Bev,

I'm sorry if you don't want to communicate by email. Because basically, that's tough shit. Stop reading now if you don't want to know what I think or know about your mom and her condition.

Right now, you are angry with me because I repeated what YOU said to your mom as she related it to me. No one expects you to care for her 24/7… that was not even suggested or discussed. What WAS discussed is what Shannon told me you had said, specifically, that there will be no finishing of the St. Pierre home bonus room because no one would ever live there. And, that Shannon would not be able to live with you if I was deceased.

If you think there was judgement or opinion included in my journal, I suggest that you re-read it. Your decisions are your business… but they do not take place in a vacuum. It is not for me to judge, and I do not even have the right to HAVE an opinion.

I have said two things consistently since this began.

1) I would tell all three of you the drop-dead honest truth about EVERYTHING. If that is not acceptable, then I will absolutely immediately and completely stop communicating with you about your mom. When Shannon asks if she is doing better or worse, I answer honestly… as I do with you guys. I WILL NOT KEEP SECRETS OR DISRESPECT ANYONE WITH LIES. Bev, if you do not want to know that she cried for the better part of two days after your conversation, then I'll share that with Brad, and if he doesn't want to know, I'll share it with my journal. But I will not obfuscate,

deny, minimize, or try to "play nice" simply because you, Bev, do not like the way it sounds. Shannon took your conversation to mean that she could never live with you, 24/7 or less, ever. If that is not true… if you did not say that… then please correct the record. BUT, if that is what you said, then live with it and don't complain about hurt feelings if you hear it repeated.

2) I have repeatedly told you both that I think Shannon should stay here until she needs a level of care that I cannot provide.

I have shared with you both the financial info of which I am certain and admitted when I was less than fully informed. I have maintained for over a year that she is best off here until her memory care and hygiene needs increase exponentially. Just last night, she woke up at 3AM and said, "I'm going to another bed."

"There's not another bed," I told her. "You're where you need to be… here with me… in your own bed." And she went quickly back to sleep.

Events such as that have increased from zero 18 months ago to at least weekly now. They will increase in both severity and frequency as we proceed. Regardless, as long as there is someone here with her… to reassure and reorient her, she is better off here, in my opinion. The alternative is some sort of nursing home that will gradually increase her care as her memory and cognitive ability decline. So, I am dedicated to the idea of keeping her right here until I DECIDE that I can no longer KEEP HER SAFE. I AM PLEASED TO DISCUSS THIS WITH YOU GUYS, BUT I AM NOT INTERESTED IN OPINIONS.

If you have facts and options to offer, then I am all ears.

But there is only one person in this discussion who supports her, makes her get dressed, takes her to doctors and shopping and Mayo and hairdressers and lunches and drives in the country,

and makes sure her friends and relatives are welcome and well-treated when they choose to visit. In short, time spent with her is the only criterion that gives anyone any say-so about these matters.

By the way, this is a 24/7 thing. Do you not realize that 24/7 care is exactly what she receives from me, NOW? And for the last two years?

Brad, as for your proposed visit, I hope you can come – you are always welcome. I think my journal may have led you to believe that Shannon is in worse shape than she is. She is probably a couple of years away from needing nursing home care. She is alert about half of the time.

(Note: this continued for a page or two. It's not relevant now and may not have been relevant even then. I'll save you the time - it is no longer important. The point is that I was as angry as I ever get about anything. SO angry that I feel it even now, welling up inside as I type.)

My concern about Bev's lack of concern go back a long way.

It began when we considered buying a travel trailer last summer. We hoped to place it in Jackson for a few months a year - so that Shannon could spend more time with Bev. I scrapped the idea when Bev told us that she MIGHT be able to spend one weekend a month with her in the trailer. Even if we bought Shannon to her, Bev could spare only one weekend a month! I cancelled the purchase.

I finished my message with the following:

"Look, guys, I am a bottom-line person. And here is the bottom line. I am your mom's husband and power of attorney. You are each secondary power of attorneys, and your power commences when mine is revoked. There are two events that could lead to that…my death or our divorce. I do not intend to hasten either, and you can count on me fighting like a caged panther if either is encouraged by either of you.

David"

December 25, 2022

Shannon told me not to email with either Bev or Brad. Then, of course, both emailed me.

Several days ago, I inquired with two local nursing facilities about their costs and their offers of home care services. Those home care services are essential to me. They can sit with her for an hour or a weekend. They can provide hygienic and minor medical care. I could take off for an afternoon or longer. So, after talking with these folks, I mentioned it to Shannon, and she wanted to drive by one of them. We did. Drove by, drove around, never stopped, and talked to no one. So, later, Shannon tells Bev, "We looked at a couple of nursing homes today" and Bev freaked. She writes to me asking if I have changed my prognosis about the two-to-five-year time frame. Did something happen? So, I wrote back to her and emphasized that nothing had changed. Shannon and Bev communicate frequently but not very effectively. Shannon is "devastated" by the idea of a nursing home… and Bev freaks. Shannon is never hungry… she is always "starving." Never chilly… always "freezing to death." One might think that Bev and Brad would have figured out that their mom is prone to hyperbole.

Anyway, enough of that. The real issue is Shannon. She handled the pre-Christmas invasion very well, though she got in a fight with Bev over an inappropriate comment that Shannon made.

Still, it was a relaxing but chaotic time. Everyone was well-fed, and everyone left. Moreover, Shannon's memory is declining so quickly that it is hard to keep track. She searches for her phone, her glasses, the TV remote, and the right words constantly. I feel SO bad for her. She has reported four major hallucinations in the last three days.

December 27, 2022

Last night, there was a noteworthy development in Shannon's illness. I was watching TV, and she was sleeping at about 10PM. She awoke and came to me.

She asked, "Where are we?"

I answered, "We are in our home in The Village. In Arkansas."

She seemed bewildered and asked, "Are you sure?"

"Yes, Babe. You are safe in your own home."

"Well, what day is Jean (the housekeeper) coming?"

"Day after tomorrow, Wednesday."

"How can that be… today is Tuesday."

"No, honey. Today is Monday. Look at the TV. Monday Night Football is on."

"That must be a re-run. I KNOW today is Tuesday.

This went on for a while…at least ten minutes. She then asked Alexa, "Alexa, what day is today?" And Alexa replied, "Today is Monday, December 26, 2022."

Shannon's head dropped to her knees, and she began to cry. "I am SO sick of this. This being confused ALL the time. When is Jean coming?"

"Day after tomorrow," I answer.

"So, Thursday."

"No, babe. Jean comes on Wednesday."

This went on for a while, and I went to bed with her. My hip is suffering from sciatica, and it's hard to stay in one position very long, but I held her in my arms until she returned to sleep, and then I quietly slipped back to the den.

Her confusion is progressing faster than I anticipated. But her normal facilities… housework, hygiene, eating… that is all good. She is talking about suicide again. Determined to never see the inside of an assisted care unit, she talks of poisons and guns. Of course, the guns are hidden away and unloaded, and she does not have the ability to load or shoot one, anyway. And she cannot drive to a pawn shop to buy a simple revolver. BUT I do have codeine in the house for my own aches. I have hidden it.

Last night's events were, I choose to believe, impermanent. The disease waxes and wanes. Good days and bad. Good weeks and bad. Last night was an outlier, I choose to believe.

December 28, 2022

Today, I called Belvedere Nursing Home in Hot Springs. I talked to Kelly, who patiently explained the financial side of nursing home care. Medicare will not pay for long-term assisted care living. That is Private Pay (or Medicaid), and the cost is over $9,000 per month at Belvedere. Medicaid will pay for long-term care if the patient is qualified financially… meaning that they have no assets, and medically, meaning that she has enough physical and mental needs. Shannon is very close, now I think, to meeting the mental criteria. I've told Bev and Brad that I THOUGHT Medicare would absorb some of the cost of assisted care living… but it will not. I now know that it is either all or nothing. If she needs care and has no resources, Medicaid will pay. If not, if she needs only minor care or a safe place to stay, no help.

The bottom line is this: if I want Shannon to be comfortable and safe, she has to stay here in our home until I can no longer take care of her hygienic and safety needs. When that time approaches, we will shop for a permanent facility. I now expect that to be in 2025. But I could be wrong, it might be next year.

She is more confused than ever. Last night, sleepless because of my sciatic hip, I met her in the kitchen at 4:00AM. She asked what time it was, and I said, “Four o’clock.” She asked, “AM or PM.” It was 100% dark. This morning, after I had fallen asleep at about 5AM, she woke me at 7AM. She had awakened earlier and canceled a doctor’s appointment that was scheduled for 2:30PM. Now, she has changed her mind and wants to reinstate the appointment but is too embarrassed to call them herself. I called, and they were happy to reinstate. While I was talking to the appointment clerk, Shannon was talking in my ear, insisting that I explain to the clerk why she had canceled the appointment so early in the day. Of course, that was not important at all, the clerk did not care, she was happy to reinstate it as the slot was open.

My sciatic injection is scheduled for Friday, and I cannot wait for that day. I had an appointment scheduled with an attorney for elder-care advice on Thursday, and the law office called today to “reschedule” which meant waiting two weeks. I told them to never mind.

December 29, 2022

After writing yesterday, I went to bed, needing rest, before driving Shannon to her doctor in Little Rock this morning. We were set to wake up at 6AM. At 11PM Shannon woke me up, asking me to go out on the deck and force her aunts to leave. After calming her down, she laid down in my bed to sleep. At 1AM she woke me again, saying it was time to get dressed and go to the doctor. "That's five hours from now," I told her, and she went back to sleep. I stayed up.

At the appointment, Shannon complained about pain in basically every part of her body. Sharp instant headaches. Sharp pains in her neck. Both hands, both knees, both feet, her stomach.

(It reminded me of an old joke. An old farmer went to a doctor, and the doctor asked, "Why are you here?"

With his index finger, the farmer pointed to a small spot on his ribcage. The doctor asked, "Is that where it hurts?"

The farmer replied, "No, this is the only spot on my body that DOES NOT HURT. Make the rest of me feel like it feels.")

And hallucinations! She told the doctor that she hallucinates several times a minute. Usually, seeing birds or rats. THAT is certainly no joke.

After arriving home around 2PM, I immediately went to sleep in the recliner. By 5PM, she had awakened me twice more. The second time, she told me that she had taken two Seroquel tablets instead of one. She's OK, of course, and I am hoping to get some sleep before getting up at 5:30AM to drive, again, to Little Rock for my epidural tomorrow morning. I would love to leave Shannon here, sleeping in her bed, but I cannot chance leaving her alone.

She just came in and asked, "Where are Bev's dogs?"

"With Bev," I said

"Where is Bev?"

"In Jackson," I answered.

"Oh, ok."

Tonight, I got a text from Shannon's therapist. She suggested I place a whiteboard in Shannon's bedroom where she can write down the day of the week, appointments, and other notes. GREAT idea. I will do that, for sure. She also recommended The Caring Place in Hot Springs. It's an adult daycare for dementia patients. Reviews are varied. I'm gonna give it a look.

I have decided to never again be intimate with Shannon. Not that it matters. We haven't been intimate in the three years since the pandemic. But I want it on the record now because I sense that Shannon is likely to soon lose the ability to legally consent.

Chapter 5
2023
Deepening Dismay

I was so much older then, I'm younger than that now.
Bob Dylan

January 2, 2023

This is a good time to write. Shannon's hallucinations and strange behavior now occupy at least 60% of her time. She frequently cannot tell night from day - often mistaking 9PM tonight for tomorrow morning… even though it is dark outside.

Last Friday, I decided that I simply had to make up with Bev and Brad. They are both wrong about this entire thing, but just like when Shannon is wrong about the night and day, arguing does me no good. So, I sent Bev a text, and tonight at 6PM she, Brad and I conferenced.

Yesterday, I called Charlie Grau to ask for his advice. As usual, he had some good ideas. Two were all I needed. After the necessary apologies and agreement that we all want the same for Shannon: safety, comfort, and security in her last years, we got down to business. With all that set up, I asked, “How do you guys see Shannon spending the next five years. What is YOUR plan.” Crickets. Neither of them had an idea. I then explained the economics of managed care… about ten grand a month for assisted care plus extra charges for locking up the wanderers, which Shannon surely is. I then asked, again at Charlie’s suggestion, “If I died tomorrow, what would you do?” Neither had an answer for that. It became apparent that neither of them had researched the issue as I had nor even thought it through. Neither was ready for what was to come. I am not sure that I am ready for it. But it is coming either way, and at least I know what I do not know.

January 20, 2023

Ten days ago we went to UAMS for Shannon’s bone density scan. On leaving, I stepped off an unseen curb and fell, face first, in the parking garage. Hit my head HARD and lost consciousness for a moment. Passersby called for an ambulance, but I shook myself off and decided to let Shannon drive me home. She did, bitching all the way about how I probably have a concussion. I DID get one heck of a shiner.

Down to business. Shannon has had two episodes lately. I define an “episode” as a sudden attack of tremors, aches, stomach pains, vomiting, and tears. Shannon is completely freaked out by them, in addition to being horribly frustrated by the entire thing. I’m impotent here. There’s nothing I can do except sit with her, comfort her, and tend to her with cold wipes and water. Her trembling is something to see. Her right arm and left leg vibrate at an amplitude of about two inches. Huge violent tremors. Scary to watch. Even more scary is the idea that they may become more frequent as the disease advances. I am on record saying that she could probably stay with me in this house for two more years. I'd hate to be wrong about that, but one never knows. If this happened every day, I don't think I could deal with it.

January 21, 2023

Mary Vance, our classmate at Woodlawn High School in the sixties, and Shannon's lifelong friend, died yesterday. She was an Alzheimer's patient, and her death had been expected. Shannon dictated the following to me for Facebook:

"With great sadness, I must say "Goodbye" to my oldest friend, Mary Ellen Vance Smith. We were placed in the same crib at Southside Baptist Church in 1950 when we were just a few months old and were inseparable friends through our childhoods. We spent many summer afternoons together at the Cedar Grove Swimming Pool and played thousands of games of Jacks. As adults, we were attendants at one another's weddings. I will miss her forever."

March 1, 2023

I must tell the story of Shannon's new drug – Nuplazid.

Prescribed by her Neurologist, Dr. Hillary Williams, this is an **expensive** drug. The UAMS pharmacist got involved, the first 14 pills were shipped immediately. In the next week we were contacted by the manufacturer, CVS Corporate, and a group that provides grants to patients for the co-pay. Our co-pay should be $1500 monthly, but they covered it for six months. Now, I know that these companies are seeking widespread adoption of the drug. There are about 5,800,000 dementia patients in the U.S. Huge market. IF the drug was priced at a price with a $1000 deductible, I would buy it, no problem. With Medicare, that means a total price of about $5000 per month. Supposing an adoption rate of ten percent, that would be 580,000 patients, and that would be thirty-five BILLION dollars annually. With revenues like that in sight, they can give away a lot of free pills.

AMAZING DRUG. This was prescribed to combat hallucinations. It worked for that, and everything else, too. I mean, Shannon stopped crying. She stopped staying in bed all day. She gets up, gets dressed, and wants to go places. She has driven me into town and simply been a wonderful companion… much like our motorhome days. I have my wife back! For a while at least, we are laughing and joking and poking fun at one another. I know that it will not last. This drug doesn't cure the disease, but it is great, for now, at managing the symptoms. Sooner or later, this progressive illness will catch up with the medication… we are still in for a LONG and trying time. But jeez, it is a nice break.

Today, I had a Teladoc appointment with Dr. Russel Tynes of Shreveport, LA. He reviewed all of my meds and explained a lot to me. This is one smart doctor who is not averse to "just talking" for an hour or so. SMART, and truly up to date.

Today, I will go to UAMS for appointments with two doctors. One is watching out for my kidneys, the other my heart. I think I will seek most of my heart care there. Just seems to make sense.

February 19, 2023

Shannon is still doing well, but a little less well than last week. She notices it, too. She asked if I thought the effects of Nuplazid, the new drug, were lessening. I told her the truth… I'm not sure. Well, that IS the truth.

April 11, 2023

Shannon is slipping more quickly. Really. Confused all of the time, gets pissed off at me very easily. I knew that the new med would not work for long, and sure enough, it has already faded.

I angered Bev again. Last winter, I asked her and her brother to take care of Shannon for two weeks this summer, which would allow me to go to Alaska to see my daughter, Macy. After visiting Bev this weekend, Shannon told me that Bev wasn't going to help. So, of course, I got pissed and sent the following email to her and Brad.

> "Bev and Brad,
>
> Y'all probably know that my 73rd birthday is just a couple of days away. Insurance actuaries estimate that this gives me about nine more years. I've been thinking about this a lot because my lifespan influences Shannon. I suppose the greatest influence it has on me is that it limits the number of times that I will see my kids. I told my old friend Lyn Anderson I had calculated that I would see each of them no more than ten more times.
>
> Lyn said, "That's unacceptable. If they cannot come to you, you have to go to them."
>
> I replied, "My responsibility to Shannon will not allow that."
>
> "Figure something out," Lyn said.
>
> And that is why I came to you guys in December… to help me figure something out. Trust me on this… I truly wish that I did not need your help. But I cannot see how Shannon can travel with me to Denver, Lake Elsinore, CA, or Fairbanks. She was exhausted after a day and a half in Jackson this past weekend. Last summer, we traveled to Virginia Beach on the first leg of a two-week trek to Massachusetts. She gave up after five days, and I brought her home. She is

quite ill today and hardly left her bed. I am devoted to her comfort, yet I think it very unfair to deprive myself and my children of the last few visits with one another.

Now, here we are, four months after I asked you guys to put your heads together and figure out a way to take care of your mother for a measly two weeks and after Shannon told me about a conversation this weekend, it is apparent to me that you guys have not worked on it at all. My choices here are extremely limited. I can go to see my daughter if I hire a 24/7 caretaker for Shannon, or if you guys step up. At this time, Shannon is very disturbed because she has no answers, no workable ideas, and she wants SO much for me to go, but she knows that such a trip is impossible for her.

This is a big deal to me. It is not just this trip, but several more. As I said - Denver and California, and not just one each. We need a system… a workable plan that we can use and reuse over these next few years. I think that Shannon will require full-time care in a couple of years. That will give me more opportunities, but then again, I will also have less time- two years will have gone by.

When this began two years ago, each of you offered to help me "in any way you can." This is no longer a theoretical construct. It is you and me and Shannon… and it is now.

David"

Bev reacted quite, ah, enthusiastically. She is very defensive and considers many discussions as attacks. Brad emailed me and explained that he and Bev have been working it out and that he will be here to watch over Shannon on July 17th. Macy says that's good! And we are all set except for plane tickets. I wish that I had known they were working on it… I went off like a firecracker when it was not necessary. I should recognize that when I get information like that from Shannon, it is likely incorrect. In fairness, they COULD have told me, you know.

April 20, 2023

Today, we made another trip to see the doctors in Little Rock. The dermatologist said that Shannon's head itch was just dandruff and prescribed nothing. Then we saw Nurse Practitioner Rachel and Sam, the pharmacist who arranged for the Nuplazid. Both were very interested in the efficacy of the drug. When I remarked that its effects seemed to be declining, both nodded knowingly. Now, I had been thinking about this, and I concluded that one of two things was happening. Either she was acclimating to the drug, or the disease was catching up with the drug. The young professionals agreed that the latter was the probable reason. That's terrible news. Shannon took the news very well… so well that I am afraid that she does not understand what it means. Her confusion and hallucinations are on the rise again… almost back to pre-Nuplazid days. It's very hard to watch… and so much harder for her.

May 2, 2023

Tonight, I am overcome by a sadness deeper than any I have ever felt.

Gerri Hayes, the mother of my good friend Gary, died three days ago. Shannon and I planned to go to her services tonight and tomorrow morning. I had promised we would attend. But we could not. Shannon had the worst day of her disease today. It started early this morning with a case of constipation. She sat on the toilet, straining, for three hours. I was giving her laxatives and softeners – to no avail. She strained for so long that her rectum began to cause her unbearable pain. She thought she had hemorrhoids, and we went to Urgent Care. They said, "No, you don't. Go take MiraLAX, drink more water, and eat fiber." This evening, after the inevitable bowel movement, she became essentially incontinent. I say "essentially" because the cause was simply the residual laxatives in her system, but the result was the same. She soiled her clothes twice and her bed once. Tonight, she is sleeping on the floor beside the bathroom door. To make matters worse, she has been terribly confused all day. The hallucinations have returned with a vengeance, and she asked me at least a dozen times if we have a guest staying with us. Times and dates overwhelm her. She wants very badly to go to Arizona to attend her granddaughter Sierra's graduation in late May. It is shaping up to be a ten-day trip, and I am concerned that she cannot stand the strain. At the speed at which this thing is progressing, I am beginning to doubt my estimate of three more years in this home. Twice today Shannon mentioned that we need to begin looking for a place for her. Whenever she mentions this, I think that she is doing so out of her own embarrassment or a desire to lessen my load. I patiently explain that our plan must be to keep her here for as long as possible. She will be more comfortable here. More secure. More time with me. Upon hearing this again, for the tenth time, she agrees… and then forgets and brings it up again. I will need help, and I can only afford to do that if we win the lawsuit. Jesus, this is frightening.

May 8, 2023

Damn! This is just misery. Shannon needs some things, but she wants a lot more. Get this: she officially announced that we need to get a new car. Balancing the money is a real job these days. The lawsuit is going to take a lot. I have paid thirty grand in advance, and I have access to another twenty grand – which is probably necessary. I simply cannot run out of money with a winning case still in court.

There is this running disagreement or whatever it is with Bev. I love Bev, and I will bet that I appreciate her talents more than anyone in her own family. But here's the deal. Bev does not seem to accept that her mom is dying. She caused a huge kerfuffle when she said that Shannon could not stay with her, in her home, when Shannon needs help. (If I was gone and Shannon had not declined far enough to require 24/7 care.) I KNOW, with all my heart, that Bev would do whatever was necessary to take care of Shannon. It could not last long IF Bev was required to intervene. The need for her to take care of Shannon would not be a long-term commitment. I doubt that Bev has considered this – that Shannon will only last a few months after she fades into 24/7 land.

This is what would have to happen to require Bev to dive in.

1. I must die. It would be helpful if I left some cash or income for Shannon, which I probably can… but, just say for now that I leave her penniless except for cars and sellable stuff.

2. Shannon would have to be still able to care for herself, but not really… she cannot take care of herself NOW.

3. So, IF Shannon did not meet the qualifications for Medicaid, she would need supervision, not total care. For a couple of years at the most, as her condition declines to the point where Medicaid kicks in.

So, I KNOW that Bev would help her own mother. Brad, too. Bev has a tender part of her mind that is triggered by any thought or suggestion that she is not a "good daughter." OF COURSE she is a good daughter. Damn. So, this happened at Christmas time. Bev and Shannon were on the deck talking, after dark. Bev busts into the house, aflame with anger. Shannon had mentioned that Bev's fever sensations might be related to menopause. And Bev freaked. Now, her mom is gonna say a LOT of inappropriate things… one cannot take it personally. I would have been gone a long time ago if I took it personally.

Shannon calls my name at least fifty times a day. Usually, it's like,

“Daaavvvee?”

“Yeah, what’s up?”

“Have you seen my phone?”

“Yeah, it’s on the coffee table.”

“What?”

“IT'S ON THE COFFEE TABLE!”

“OK.”

But sometimes, it is:

“Daaavvveee? I want to rearrange the furniture in the den.”

“WHAT THE HELL? REALLY? Jesus, why?”

(Forget the lawsuit. Overlook the fact that she is dying while I am fighting for breath and our financial life. Forget all of that, we need to rearrange the furniture.)

And away we go. That goes on constantly. This financial fight, with the lawsuit and all, would be a lot easier with her cooperation. She gets very upset with herself when she screws up. Last night, she thought she had found a third C-PAP device in her bedroom. Not possible. She had found her miniature heater. It’s small, white, and electrical. Must be a C-PAP, right?

That is not the problem. The problem is that she gets upset. Cries. Stays that way for half an hour. Or two hours. Then, I hear, “Daaavvvee?”

May 13, 2023

I have a new CPA for taxes. In response to her question about medical expenses, I sent this:

"Shannon has Lewy Body Dementia. It is a terminal Alzheimer's/Parkinson's "hybrid" that is just relentless. And, you're correct… she takes two thousand dollars a month in pills, but Medicare gets most of that. We are sort of struggling to get along with it… difficult because it is progressive, and every week brings new challenges. I'm just a passenger, attempting to keep her warm and safe as this ship sails over the horizon."

We leave for Arizona in a few days. We made this trip a couple of years ago, and it taxed me down to zero. Shannon was better then than now and handled that trip easily. But we stayed at altitude, on Mt. Humphreys… maybe seven thousand feet, and I had trouble breathing. In fact, I was so miserable that we stayed only one night, with me sipping on the oxygen can every few minutes. On the way out of town, Shannon noticed a series of trails that led up the nearby mountainside. "Oh, we should take those trails to the top of the mountain," she announced. Sigh.

This time, we will be staying in Sedona, one of my favorite places. Sedona is within easy striking distance, and its elevation is only five thousand feet.

May 23, 2023

We are in Santa Fe tonight. Left home Sunday afternoon, following a quick visit from Shannon's friends Dawn and Eric from Dallas. They're nice folks and Shannon gets revved up by visitors. We drove to Oklahoma City on the first day, and to Tucumcari, New Mexico, on Monday. Tomorrow, we spend most of the day and the night with more of Shannon's friends, Jane Brennan et ux (that's realtor talk for 'and husband'), who live here in Santa Fe. We drive to Sedona on Thursday. Brad's daughter's high school graduation is Friday. We are staying in Sedona… 30 miles away and 2000 feet lower for my breathing… which is much better, by the way.

Shannon has had a couple of meltdowns on the trip, so far. She gets stressed out so easily… even with me right there to assure her that all is well, and we are on vacation to see her son and grandkids. Her stress is followed by periods of tearful frustration and then a period of recovery. She is actually doing well. Oh, sometimes she loses her glasses and phone twice during one lunch, but we always find them.

Each month, I join a group therapy/sharing session via Zoom with several others from all over the state. Last week, they asked me what I was doing to cope. Well, nothing. I don't try to take time off or go to strip clubs or drink too much… what do I do? Then I realized what I really do. I have a good attitude. Not to brag, it's not really a *good* attitude… just a mature one. When Shannon does something goofy or inappropriate, I let it roll off. If she changes her mind three times before we get to the restaurant she chose, that's OK. I told the group this, and they were astonished. "How do you keep your cool like that? We know about the frustrations… how do you cope?"

"It's not about me!" I tell them. It could have been me, I tell them. I am the lucky one, I say. When Shannon has a problem, it is not about me. It's about only Shannon. It was like that with my mom, sixty years ago, and with my sister forty years ago. Both were bi-polar. Both sometimes went off their meds. Both required occasional hospitalizations, and both required constant attention after dad's death in 1983. I only needed to remind myself, frequently, that I drew the longer straw in the gene lottery. Which would I rather be - the helpless or the helper? That single thought has been a foundation for strength when times get really tough. It could have been me.

July 16, 2023

The following message was left for Bev and Brad before I departed for Alaska to visit Macy.

“Hi. I wanted to visit with you about your mom’s drugs. (You probably know all of this. I’m not talking down to you – I just want to warn you about her foibles and hopefully enable you to dig deep into your well of patience.)

She has two weeks’ worth of pills prepacked into those little seven-day containers. She has a total of six containers - three for each week; morning, mid-day, and bedtime. Now, she will, without supervision, mix them up. It’s a good idea to ask her, at least twice a day, if she had her morning pills… her mid-day pills… her evening pills. CHECK them. She will often miss a dose, and then get confused and frustrated and even tearful about her failing ability to keep them… or anything else… straight.

Her most apparent forgetfulness shows up in confusion about which day it is, what time it is, etc. Expect her to ask if there are other people in the house… especially after waking. She dreams that granny is here, then wonders where granny is sleeping, if she is hungry, that sort of thing. Please try to be gentle but firm with her. She’ll ask you the same thing four times… apologizing each time.

"When are we leaving?”

“We are going at 6PM.” (Please do not add “I already told you.”) She knows that but cannot remember and hates herself for it. She had a little bit of a panic attack last night and woke me at 3AM to help her calm down. She had dreamed that we could not get all the suitcases into the car, and it took half an hour for her breathing to return to normal.

She won’t eat anything (almost anything) that you cook. Expect a lot of pizza and hamburgers. And Lean Cuisine. Trust me… I have given up trying. She has developed a fondness for throwing food away. Please let her throw away whatever she wants. Wrinkled tomatoes, anything in the fridge that’s past its expiration date, that stuff. When she asks, "Can I throw this away?" do not even discuss it. "Mom, throw away anything you want. Dave made that clear."

Thank you both for allowing me this visit with my daughter, and the break from the responsibility. What I am telling you might sound simple and elementary... does he think we are idiots? No, of course not. Just please, do not express impatience or anger with her... she can really close up on you quickly. And watch the meds.

Good luck, and thanks again.

David"

August 10, 2023

I've been putting off writing for a couple of weeks. Alaska got in the way, and I've been lazy. There's not much to write about. Her mood continues to darken, and she is confused by every number in the universe.

September 18, 2023

Shannon is now declining visibly. I mean that every day is a little worse. Just a little, but it is definitely worse and readily apparent. At this moment, she has strep throat and feels terrible. That certainly exacerbates her dementia. She never knows what day it is. She went to see her primary care physician this week, and did not know what month it is. EVERY day, she awakens and asks where our guests are sleeping. Usually, she is concerned about Brad or Bev, but it is often her late mother or sister Patti. We are looking for a new car and she stays confused. This and similar mental vacancies are far more common now than previously. I can detect a difference this month. I have taken over the meds completely, and her doctor told her not to drive.

We are planning on traveling to Shreveport on September 3. We'll watch LSU v Florida State that night, stay with Gary and Patricia Hayes Sunday and Monday night, then go to a pre-trial hearing at the Bossier Parish Courthouse. I HOPE this hearing is where the action begins. I am 100% convinced that we should win, but that's why we have trials. And card games, car races, football. You never know until you do it.

October 2, 2023

It has been a while, and there is a ton to write about. My ability to keep this journal up to date is declining as my need for rest increases.

Our trip to Shreveport did not include seeing Gary and Patricia. Patricia was hospitalized, and we do not yet know if she is OK.

We are leaving in two days to fly to Denver. We will see my son Hank, his wife Mandy, whom I have written about, and the Eagles in concert. I have four tickets in the cheap seats. I can tell that Hank and Mandy are excited. We will get there on Wednesday the fourth and return on the ninth.

Shannon's condition is going down rapidly now. Maybe it's that up again, down again thing. But she never knows what day it is or what time it is. If we have a one-hour trip to Little Rock, and we need to be there at noon, she cannot figure out if we need to leave at 11AM or 1PM. It is scary. A few days ago, we were driving, and she screamed at me to stop. She "saw" a truck stopped sideways in the road ahead. Last night, she "saw" mice on the deck. Her hallucinations have reached a new peak and now include sounds. Three times this evening, she asked me if I was calling her. She wanted to drive to church this morning but was unable to do so and refused my offer to drive her. She is through driving, and probably will not ask again.

She has made several similar comments lately. “I cannot believe how fast this is going.” “I am so afraid of what is to come.” I hope she will reach a point where her decline is not so obvious to her. She has even said the same thing.

I am finished for tonight.

October 13, 2023

Shannon is slipping more quickly now. She never knows what day it is, often asking several times in a day. She is seeing hallucinations constantly. This morning, she asked me to see who was sitting in our car in the garage, remarked about tonight’s Halloween trick-or-treaters (that’s in two weeks, not tonight), and called out to Patti. Then she told me, while sitting in the den, that she was talking with Ethan and Addy – “They're right there on the sofa, can't you see them?”

She has awakened me three times in the last week to fix her TV or phone, both of which she is having more and more trouble using. The problems are always something that she has fouled up in settings. How she gets to that spot I cannot imagine. This is The. Saddest. Thing. I have ever seen, period.

October 16, 2023

A few days ago, Shannon and I met as we rounded a corner into the den. I stopped to hug her, and she began sobbing those long, quivering cries that have one’s shoulders jumping up and down. “I don’t want to go,” she mumbled.

Last night, she came into my bedroom to sleep. But there was very little sleep. She was vividly dreaming that she was in Bev’s former home in Texas and that Bev’s roommate was returning home soon and would catch Shannon and me in bed. She woke me to say that this VRBO we were staying in was "exactly like our house in Arkansas, all the way down to the linen closet." Sometimes, I just go along with her. When her deceased Aunt Tommie was "visiting" us last week, Shannon became concerned that Aunt Tommie had not returned from the store. "We have to go find her!"

"Yes, we will. Let's just have a bite to eat first," and she forgot about it. I learned this strategy from literature and videos on caretaking for dementia patients. The caretaker must be gentle and soothing… sometimes firm, and others totally receptive to the patient. Otherwise, the patient will shut down.

Tonight, we are prepping for a visit to Shannon's movement specialists tomorrow. Shannon is totally out of it. She thinks that we are at a VRBO in Karnack, TX, and that we cannot make it to UAMS on time. I couldn't talk her down. Until tonight, I was always able to get her to come around. Tonight… no way.

November 6, 2023

The last two weeks have been filled with Shannon's troubles. Hallucinations are so numerous and lengthy that she seems to get lost in them. She sees people from her family. They are living in the Toyota, skulking around the garage, partying on the deck… they are everywhere. I awoke at 6AM to find her outside in the front yard. It got so bad that her neurologist told us to come to the emergency room in Little Rock. We were there for thirty-six hours, and all they did was increase her script to three tabs of Seroquel daily, instead of one.

Tomorrow, I go to work on Medicaid full time. I must get this done. Bev is acting as if she has no responsibility here. She, Brad, and I had a conference call, and she kept asking me, "Can't you pay that?" whenever I mentioned any cost. I am exhausted, and I want to begin bringing in-home healthcare workers as Shannon's needs grow. And I hope to get help from Hospice, but if not, I expect Bev and Brad to help. Bev seems to think that she can simply say, "I have no money" and that will be that. She does not seem to understand that I am not tied to this by anything except my love for Shannon. I can leave Bev with the entire load if I think that is the only way to get the help Shannon needs. That would be unimaginably difficult for me. I'm the guy who hangs in there. But, I am just SO tired. Tired to the point of doubting my ability to keep her safe. So, if this does not change, I will someday soon tell Bev that I am divorcing her mother, and that she can deal with it herself. I will cry as I do so, but this simply must change. I'm not physically capable of doing it all alone for much longer.

Last year, when she asked how she could help, I had an idea. We have used a once-a-month housekeeper for a couple of years, and I have been planning on increasing that to twice monthly. The cost is seventy-five dollars per visit. So, I told Bev that I could increase that to a visit every week if she could pay for two per month – I would pay for two. She agreed immediately, it seemed like a good idea. I set it up with the housekeeper. In the next ten months, Bev sent ONE payment. Then, when I finally asked about it, she became angry with me!

We also had an agreement that she would visit us once a month. I was very pleased. Shannon would get more time with her daughter, and I would have a weekend off. I could see old friends or just check into a Holiday Inn and sleep. I think she kept her part of that agreement two times in two years. At least twice, Shannon phoned to check on her as she was traveling here on a Friday evening, and she found that she had departed only a few minutes before or not at all. On those two occasions, Shannon did what all mothers would do. "Oh, Bev, you don't have to come this weekend. I am afraid for you driving at night." And with that, Bev turned around and went back home –

presumably to another tennis tournament. It seems to me that Bev actually did not want to come and seized on the first chance to return to Jackson. Twice, I attempted to emphasize to Bev the importance of her visits to Shannon and to Bev herself. "There will come a time, I am certain, when you will look back and think of the time you left on the table and the opportunities you squandered. But it will be too late." She told me to mind my own business.

November 7, 2023

BIG NEWS

From: David

Sent: Monday, November 6, 2023 11:56:06 PM

To: 'Bev, Brad

Subject: Hospice

"A few days ago, I called our Medicare insurance agent after receiving conflicting info from different sources. She has guided us with great care through the ocean of Medicare Advantage plans to one that has served us well. She said, "David, I do not understand it, either. So, I asked for the help of a hospice company with my mother." And she recommended a woman named Cheryl from Dierksen Hospice.

I called Dierksen at 11AM today, and a representative named Jaimie Floyd called back immediately and was at our home at 12:50PM. Extremely professional with years of experience in this field. Bev, I'll text you her phone number so that you can call… she explicitly said that she welcomes all questions.

She said that many people think of Hospice as an "end of life" alternative, when it is actually much more. I can tell you that I believe these guys have it covered. We will certainly use the hospice services (you'll see why in a minute), but there are MANY companies in the business.

Hospice is the missing link to the conflicting information we have received. They are the connector to Medicare, and when the time comes, to Medicaid. As I have written, Medicare will not pay for long-term care. And Medicaid will not pay for the treatment of diseases. HOWEVER, Medicare will pay for all of the services of Hospice as long as we are not seeking aggressive treatment. NOTHING OUT OF POCKET!!! My understanding is that Medicare will pay for home health care, equipment, supplies, and 5 days at a time of "respite care" which means that Shannon can stay in a hospital for up to five days while I get a rest. They will put a nurse, priest, or health care worker in the home AT NO COST TO US during Shannon's decline. When Shannon needs a 24/7 facility, they will offer us options for nearby homes that accept Medicaid and then handle the admission and payment paperwork. They will send a social worker to our home with 24-hour notice to explain further, discuss financial planning, set down a plan, answer questions, etc. They have an RN who lives here in Hot Springs Village. They were recommended by my insurance agent. They know their stuff. Oh, Jaimie told us to call her or her partner if we have questions. Her partner's name is Cheryl.

If you detect a tone of relief and elation in this email, it is correct. I KNEW that we were missing something, and this is it.

David"

November 17, 2023

It has been an eventful week here in the land of LBD. First, we are now signed up for hospice service. They WILL NOT pay for the home health care needs that I foresee. I'm annoyed that they did not level with us in advance on this, though it would not have affected our decision. So far, we have had a sales nurse, an intake nurse, our actual nurse (who lives in HSV and will visit weekly), and a social worker visit us at home. And a priest/pastor/preacher/ called today for an appointment. So, we are in the system, and we shall see how it works.

In other news, I have been kicked out of the dementia support group with which I had attended three meetings. The director of the group sent me an email saying that I had made inappropriate comments in their meetings. I have no idea what she was referring to. This is the email she sent to me:

> From: Kathy Packard
>
> Sent: Thursday, November 16, 2023 8:18 AM
>
> To: David Legan
>
> Subject: Caregiver Support group
>
> "David,
>
> The caregivers who attend our support groups need the support of the group to face the daily challenges of caregiving. I became concerned after you attended the Hot Springs support group and made inappropriate comments to Lee Kathryn. I cannot and will not tolerate that behavior. Yesterday, you made another inappropriate comment regarding your marriage. Our mission in our support groups is to support and encourage a loving relationship between the caregiver and the care receiver and to provide resources to ease the burden of caregiving.
>
> I know this is a very difficult time for you, and I believe you would benefit from individual counseling, which we do not provide. Due to

the inappropriate comments, you will not be invited back to the support group.

Respectfully,

Kathy"

Kathy Packard, MS, M.Ed, LPC, CADDCT, CDCM, CFRDT, CDP

Executive DirectorCenter on Aging, Inc.Hot Springs, AR 71901

I mailed an apology to Ms. Packard and Lee Kathryn, who I do not remember, and never heard from either again.

But check out that signature, will you? Just look at all of those letters after her name. Ms. Packard has every certification known to man, maybe using them as a backstop. My understanding is that her organization is funded by Oaklawn Downs, and the gambling they host there. For my money, the annoying publication of her certifications on every email and her business card reveals a deep insecurity and/or narcissism.

I once met Soichiro Honda, the founder and then CEO of Honda Motor Co, LTD. (I also danced with Mrs. Honda… as a 22 year old Junior Representative, on the convention floor with the wife of my hero.) He was one of the finest engineers/businessmen in the world, brilliant and acknowledged as such. Guess what HIS business card said.

Soichiro Honda
Honda Motor Company, LTD
(International phone number)

Mr. Honda did not need the reassurance of a load of initials. He was not seeking power or affirmation. He was a self-made man, a spectacular success, and a temple of confidence. No sir, no certificates of accomplishment for Mr. Honda.

I realized why being booted from the dementia support group bothered me so. It bothered me because I was accused of saying something rude to one of the vendors. Several women representing various caretaking-for-a-fee companies regularly bring lunch to these meetings, and I had reportedly said something "inappropriate" to one of them. Well, that is not me. I can be a Grade A smart-ass, but I am NOT rude, and these women were nothing but nice to me. But I had told the group about one of Shannon's hallucinations, the one where she mistook our home for a VRBO. That brought a little laugh, but maybe she with all the initials, found it inappropriate.

Then, I remembered. I told the group that I had reacted to Shannon's wandering outside by adding double deadbolt locks to the two doors. Ms. Packard interrupted me to ask, "Are you not afraid of a fire, with the doors locked?" I was startled. Surely, she did not think of me as too stupid to consider and plan for that.

So, instead of arguing with her, and possibly embarrassing her in front of her group, I quipped, "Well. I have owned a home for fifty years with no fires. But, one year into this and she has escaped twice." It made sense to me and was delivered with a smile. Now, I think maybe she did not think of it as funny.

And finally, we went to a local clinic today for a blood draw. The neurologist has one bullet left in her gun… Clozapine. It is a powerful anti-psychotic and requires weekly blood tests to ensure that no harm is being done. Something about white blood cells.

Now, to Shannon. Her hallucinations are absolutely over the top. She talks to these "people" constantly. Telling them to leave, get out of here, and put her jewelry back in the box. It is far beyond frustrating… it is heartbreaking. She came to me last night and said, in a hushed whisper, “Do you have something to tell me?”

"No," I said. “What do you mean?”

She said, “When are you gonna tell me the truth about these people staying in our home?” Today, she did not remember that. Sigh.

Shannon is seeing “tribbles.” You might remember a Star Trek episode, “The Trouble with Tribbles.” They were small, spiny creatures that looked like sea urchins and multiplied quickly. At the beginning of the episode they were cute. Then, they were troublesome. Then, they were genuinely dangerous. Shannon sees them everywhere. She steps carefully to avoid them, brushes them off the couch, and shouts at them.

December 20, 2023

The Clozapine is helping a LOT with the hallucinations. I am convinced, however, that she needs to double the dosage she is getting. They control this stuff like it is an atomic weapon… weekly blood draws, and prescriptions for only 15 pills at a time. Last week, she had a meltdown in the afternoon with the next pill scheduled for the evening. I gave her an extra one that day, and she improved instantly. This drug is prescribed in strengths up to 200mg, and doctors often start with a small dosage, and plan increases as the patient adapts to it. Shannon’s dosage is only 12.5mg. I lobbied with her doctors to increase that to two a day, but they wouldn’t do it. As I write this, she is now arguing with her “visitors” and demanding that they leave the house. Damn, this is frustrating. A nurse suggested that I keep a ledger of her hallucinations. I have been doing that for over two years. In fact, you are reading it now.

This weekend, she travels to Jackson for Christmas with Bev, who will pick Shannon up here on Friday, the 22. I will then drive to Texas to see John Haigler and cousin JoAnn and stop to see Gary and Patricia Hayes (now out of the hospital) for Christmas dinner. Shannon would rather be with her daughter and son-in-law, who are not speaking to me, than me. Bev and I no longer communicate. She is impossible to talk with… almost hysterical at times… and called me a narcissist. Her husband is even worse. So, when they retrieve her, I'll haul ass. Then I will pick her up at their home without getting out of the car. It's a miserable situation, but less miserable than trying to feign it with Bev.

Merry Christmas and Happy New Year.

Chapter 6
2024
The Last Tomorrow

Likely one of us is going to spend some time alone.
Jason Isbell

January 2, 2024

Oh brother, this has become too real. We visited her newest doctor, a psychiatrist, last week. He agreed to increase the dosage of Clozapine, the new drug that seemed, at first, to reduce her hallucinations. When taking one small dose per day, she had a couple of meltdowns, which were stopped by a second dose. So, good on the doctor for listening to me and increasing the dosage. But the hallucinations are already worse than before the increase. There is no relief.

I have accepted that Shannon will not survive to year's end. Tonight, she asked me to prepare plates of food for the visitors, Holly and Addy. She asked for the key so she could let them inside. A difficult part (for me) is that she expects to discuss them with me as if they are real. Last night, she woke me at 4AM, standing beside the bed, rattling a keychain in my face and asking which of these keys would open the door so she could let them in. I was so startled that it did not anger me. Just alarmed at being awakened so suddenly to find a set of keys in my face. What if she DOES get out? I am no longer able to guarantee her safety.

What about MY safety? I once dated a woman whose mother, mentally ill, stabbed her brother to death as he slept in his bed. I think I will not fret over that. I am doing all I can, including often going without sleep, exercise, PT, etc. We are visiting a nursing home and an "at-home assistance" company tomorrow. We were approved for a grant of up to $1500 for six months of periodic "respite care" for me. (They will pay a sitter for her for a couple of hours a week.) It will take a while to take effect, but it will come in handy. We go to the psychiatrist again this week.

An old friend contacted me over the holidays to wish me a happy new year and check on Shannon. I wrote back to him:

> "Reid,
>
> I have never in my life been afraid. Oh, I have scared myself shitless on many occasions. My little Cessna over Lake Pontchartrain, race bikes all over the country, and many women have scared the bejesus out of me, but I have never been afraid. And now, now I feel the fear welling up as I never have. I'm terrified, and there is no one to help. No help is even possible. I guess this is my first ever solid contact with an unchangeable outcome. Hopelessness… now, THAT is something to be afraid of.
>
> Best,
>
> David"

January 11, 2024

News. We visited a marvelous nursing home that accepts Medicaid. Belvedere. The place is so new and well-kept that I am amazed. Shannon, too. There is a great business manager there named Brandon Autrey who promised to help us with the paperwork. We also visited a service, Right at Home, that can provide temporary hourly care through Medicaid, as well. Medicaid only reimburses them at twenty dollars per hour, and they typically charge twenty-seven dollars, so they limit adding Medicaid patients. I volunteered to pay an additional seven bucks out of pocket, so I think we have a deal.

We also visited an Elder Care attorney who was highly recommended. It was a free consultation, but I insisted on paying him two hundred dollars in cash because, as I told him, "When you see my name on caller ID, I want you to take the call with pleasure." He approved of the powers of attorney we had created three years ago and refined our knowledge of nursing home Medicaid admission procedures. One interesting fact that we did not know is that the nursing home will likely require the first month to be paid by us, out of our pocket. So, getting her accepted will cost between six and ten thousand dollars. We are therefore seriously considering the possibility of locating her somewhere else… probably Jackson, and Bev has taken on the scouting duties there. Apparently, it will be no problem to transfer her to Mississippi if we start here first, but I think the "first month private pay" might apply on the move, too. So, there is that. The only advantage of beginning at the local Belvedere facility is that she could probably gain admission more quickly than in Jackson, when the time comes, due to my expectation of personalized assistance that I have developed here.

Shannon is always at her best when talking with these people. She tours a facility as if she is looking for a spot for her mom and impresses everyone with her ability to converse. Then, back in the car, she breaks down. In fact, she spends a lot of time crying and asking such questions as "Why me?" and "What did I do to deserve this?" Absolutely heartbreaking.

Later today, we will visit her Neurologist.

January 25, 2024

The visit with Dr. Williams was "run of the mill." She is restrained and offers very little. There's nothing more to offer – she has emptied her magazine of bullets. Shannon mentioned her knee, and Dr. Williams tried to pull rank and get her the X-ray she needed, but it was late in the day, and we returned home without the X-ray.

In the last few days, we have gone twice to Little Rock. First, to a UAMS Outpatient clinic where Shannon saw a very nice Dr. Nance about her knee. She wants imaging, which we will have soon. The following day, we returned to Little Rock to see a recent addition to The Shannon Woodruff Medical Team, a young psychologist named Adam Dodd. He is an earnest and enthusiastic young man, willing to listen and kind with his advice. But he is incapable of treating Shannon's disease. I watch his eyes for a hint of his thoughts. Does he see Shannon as a feeble and dying patient? Or, as someone he can help? I have no idea, but if seeing him does anything to improve Shannon's underlying sorrow, I'm fine with it.

January 28, 2024

Oh, shit. It's been only a few days since I wrote here. Recent developments have been SO discouraging and SO time-consuming that neither my time nor energy allowed me a chance to sit down.

I am swimming in an ocean of sorrow. Shannon's hallucinations have gotten far worse, despite two doses of Clozapine per day. She is essentially living in a world of her own making. She is convinced that I know about other people staying in our home with us, and that I AM gaslighting her by refusing to name them or admit to seeing them. She says, "You KNOW they are here! You are trying to make me go crazy!" She looks me straight in the eye and accuses me of having an affair with Addy or Sierra (both teenagers within the family) or someone else. She sees images of people hiding beneath crumpled towels and napkins. She can hardly walk due to a knee bummer of unknown origin. Two doctors and their X-rays and MRIs have revealed no damage, yet her knee is swollen far beyond its normal size and hurts her constantly. I think it could be gout, and I have the most used drug for gout in my cabinet, but she will not take it, and the doctors just want more tests.

I need to talk to Brad. Texted him earlier today, but he has not answered. I need to talk to him about Shannon's nursing home. Shannon and her children must decide about where she will stay. Here in Arkansas, is one choice. Shreveport, Dallas, and Jackson are the others. Now, here's the concern. My home is in Arkansas, allowing me to visit her as often as possible. But I hope to do some traveling. Get a van and a small motorcycle and travel. Visit my kids and old friends. I have only recently begun to think about "what the hell will I do with myself?" That's the best I can come up with. So, where should Shannon stay where she can be most often visited by friends and relatives? Bev is in Jackson. Her high school friends are in Shreveport. Her adult friends are in Dallas. Some relatives, too. I am the only person in Arkansas who will visit her. But I might be gone a bit. It hurts to think of her alone, but I am losing my ability to cope, and I have no idea how I will feel with her in a nursing home.

I am going to go full tilt to get her Medicaid approval as soon as possible. She NEEDS to be in a protected place. Last night she attempted to crawl through a window in her bedroom. It is twenty feet down to the forest floor outside, and she was only stopped by accidentally stepping onto a central heating vent plate on the floor.

A problem is that sometimes she seems to be perfectly OK. We visited an elder care Attorney on January 9, and he remarked that she seems just fine. No administrator would admit her to a Medicaid-funded home if she was this alert and making jokes. But then she gets home, and she changes back. Yesterday, she insisted on going to Lowe's but then could not walk into the store.

Frustration is covering me in an avalanche of hopelessness.

February 7, 2024

Tonight, we faced the most frightening episode yet. Shannon fainted and fell to the floor, unconscious, (as I wrote about in a previous chapter.)

I finished the application for Medicaid today, and tried to deliver it to Brandon, at Belvedere Nursing Home. He was out of the office. I have an appointment with him in two days, and then I intend to walk the application through the Health and Human Services office, if they will allow it. I am no longer confident in my ability to keep her safe.

February 9, 2024

As I mentioned, Shannon has a bad knee. A seriously damaged left knee, upon which she cannot walk. This is the knee in which she had a tumor at age twenty-five or so. It was put back together, post-tumor, with steel rods and plastic concrete. It has bothered her intermittently for as long as I have known her, but this is different. It is badly swollen, and she gets around on crutches and a cane, wincing at every step. We recently made two visits to an emergency care unit of Baptist Health in Little Rock. She needs a knee replacement – nothing short of that can help. This is actually more serious than it sounds. First, my girl is in excruciating pain. Second, it is another thing to deal with. And third, it is another brick in the wall of ailments that are predicted to presage the end.

There is ANOTHER new member of Shannon's Medical Team, a psychiatrist named Dr. Kirkpatrick. He has no reservations about prescribing drugs. Don't misunderstand, he is not a "drug-slinger." However, he is willing and ready to prescribe those that he feels will help the patient. I am glad to see this. After meeting him yesterday, we did not even have to leave the building to see the psychologist, Adam Dodd. I do not attend those meetings… Shannon can talk about me (or anything else) without holding back. The truth is that there is nothing Shannon could say at this point to hurt my feelings. Or to discourage me from caring for her to the best of my ability.

February 29, 2024

The Medicaid application is in the hands of the administrator of Belvedere Nursing Home. I have also contacted a company named Helping Hands. This company can also apply for Medicaid assistance with help around the house. They think they can get approval for sixty hours a month. So, four trips of four hours each per week. That would help immeasurably. There'd be no housework, and Shannon would have someone to help her organize, dress, shower, makeup… all of that stuff!

I want to tell a short story that illustrates the conundrum I find myself facing. Two weeks ago, we went to the doctor for the fourth time about Shannon's knee. She had removed her pants and was wearing a disposable pair of shorts so the physician could examine the knee. Only a knee replacement can lessen the pain. Well, that and drugs. As Shannon began to put her pants back on, she stood on one leg and awkwardly tried to bend enough at the waist to put her other leg, which would not bend, into the pant leg. She lost her balance, of course, and I caught her. I then asked her to sit on the adjacent chair and put her pants on without risking her life. (We have had this discussion before. With only one good leg, she insists on standing on it and convoluting her body to stretch a crimped-up knee into the other pantleg.) She refused and lost her balance again with the same result. Again, I caught her and told her, more sternly this time, to sit down. She did not want to sit down in her underwear on the chair in the doctor's office, as if the seat might have a virus. I then told her to sit. She did, and the pants went on easily. But there was tension in the air.

It was drizzling rain as we left the office. Our car was parked precisely facing the door, across two driving lanes of the parking lot, facing us. It was thirty feet away. Shannon was confused, barely able to hold her balance, and leaning on her cane, spinning in circles in the drizzle and asking, "Where is the car? Where is the car?" (I should have been steadying her, but she had wandered away as I returned the wheelchair we used to take her outside.) I began to call out to her, "Turn around." The traffic drowned my voice, and as I walked toward her, I raised my voice. "Turn around!" I said, pointing.

On the way home, she reprimanded me for raising my voice to her, twice, in a matter of minutes. I was flustered and almost became defensive. But I held my tongue and thought about it instead. She was right. I should have been more gentle. And thinking some more, I began to realize the insane difficulty of my situation. I cannot leave her by herself. We are together 24/7. She is constantly in need. She will call me twenty times (at least) every day to find her phone, fix her TV remote, bring her pills, take her to Sonic, start the dishwasher, make her bed… on and on. Not big stuff, but not within her abilities, either. So, I get no break. I have not had an adult conversation in months. I talk with therapists and doctors. I speak with my attorney. And I get a few calls a month from my children and a few friends. I

AM physically and emotionally exhausted. The inevitable result is frustration. I'm on pins and needles constantly. There is simply no way that I can maintain a gentle, calm posture every second of every day. And that is the conundrum – she needs care at a level that I am simply too exhausted to provide. And the harder I try, the more exhausted I become.

Shannon has mentioned almost daily that she wants to go to a nursing home. Today, I received word that the Medicaid application is now in the possession of Helping Hands, the company that may provide her with in-home care. If that works out, we will have a chance to spend a few more months together. In two days, I'll be talking with Bev and Brad. We shall see.

This week, we saw Shannon's PCP, Dr. Lau, a bright woman with a great human touch, and we saw the psychologist again. I had two appointments with physicians, myself, but those are unimportant.

March 6, 2024

Shannon is in the hospital. The Geriatric Behavior clinic at Baptist Hospital. Last night, they took her from the emergency room, wearing nothing but a hospital gown and carrying NO personal effects. She is miserable. I did not get to see her today. Visiting "hours" are only one hour, and I had two doctor's appointments that kept me away. I'll see her tomorrow. Last Saturday was unbelievable. She awoke in a hallucination and stayed in it for 48 hours. She fell three times. She hallucinated about a wedding to be held in our house… where is everyone gonna sleep… can we feed them all… where is Brad… is Bev sleeping with her… is Addie sleeping with me. She said she wanted to go to the hospital, and I took her there the next day. Bev is definitely taking an interest. More on that later- I am too tired right now.

March 28, 2024

Shannon was discharged today from the Behavioral Unit at Baptist Hospital. She was in NO WAY prepared for or capable of living either alone or with me in our home. These are the saddest days of my life. She has been approved for admission to The Blossoms at Midtown Little Rock and will enter into their care next week. We intend to enjoy, as much as possible, our last few days in our home. Unless there are extraordinary developments in the next few days, I will not be writing. I want to comfort her, to hold her hand, and allow her to fall asleep in my arms. So, I will not have either time or inclination to write anything.

A few days ago I brought Shannon's cell phone home from the Behavorial Unit. While stashing it on the foyer table, it beeped a notification and spying, I opened it to discover a group text-chat to which Shannon was supposed to be a party. Bev, her husband, Brad, and cousin Melonie were chatting, and I was the subject.

Melonie said Shannon should "get away from his drunk ass."

Bev's husband remarked "He is the devil!"

Chad was silent.

Bev wrote, "And now he is threatening to… wait, he has Shannon's phone… he might be on it right now!"

Bev was about to tell them that I had threatened to divorce Shannon. I doubt that she would have told them that I made the threat out of exhaustion with being Shannon's *sole caretaker*. That, except for two weeks when they cared for her in 2023, neither Bev nor Brad had come to care for her, or sent even a few dollars to help in her care. Melonie, too. Bev would certainly not repeat my words; "Bev, if you are unwilling to contribute to her care, I will be forced to divorce her and leave you with the entire load."

None of these four were in town or visiting Shannon, yet all of them gathered in cyberspace to insult me and demonstrate their cluelessness. Thinking of this now, it should have been heart-breaking. It should have left me in quivering confused anger. It did not. I am numb from hopelessness and sleeplessness and the overwhelming burden of my responsibility. They do not know. They are ignorant. I wasn't angry just as one would not be angry with a young child who could not solve an algebra problem.

April 3, 2024

Shannon entered The Blossoms at Midtown Nursing Home today. I drove her there and carried her clothing and bedding to her room on the second floor. I stayed with her for an hour, then we went to lunch. After lunch, we returned to her room, and I did what I could to make her feel at home. Of course, my actions were woefully inadequate. Returning to my car, I drove gently away from the parking place and steered into the adjacent parking lot, stopped the car, and wept.

April 7, 2024

Charlie is here! He came up from Shreveport, making his annual spring swing from Florida. He will return to Virginia Beach in a few days, after we have bashed our guitars through a load of old-time country songs. To Charlie and me, John Prine and Jackson Browne are newcomers.

April 8, 2024

Today was the day of the ECLIPSE! Little Rock was in the dead center of the path. I pulled Shannon out of the Blossoms, and she, Charlie, and I watched every minute of it, transfixed, from the Chipotle parking lot. For a few minutes, we escaped. I am really glad that she was able to see Charlie, and Charlie said more than once that he would forever remember his last contact with her.

April 10, 2024

Charlie is gone, and both Brad and Bev are flying in this weekend. I visited Shannon after seeing a physician earlier. She does NOT like the nursing home and demands to be taken home. I sometimes ask, "To which home?" and she might answer, "Dallas" or "Just forget it." This might make me sound cruel, it might seem that I am teasing her. But, if she were ever to answer, "Hot Springs Village, Silly," I would help her pack. That would be a miracle, and it will not happen.

I HATE this… this resignation. This acceptance that I am really losing Shannon. In fact, I think I already have lost her. I do think she is aware of my presence, but still, it seems that she often does not recognize me. I take her to lunch almost every day. That assures me that she IS eating, at least something. Her physical condition is just terrible. She does manage to enter and exit the car, but only with physical help and instruction.

At heart, I am a "fourth-quarter guy." I grew up playing and watching football, and I believe that my team, the one that is two touchdowns behind in the fourth quarter, will still pull off a last second victory. I believe in the last-minute, come-from-behind miracle. Every cell in my body recoils as I try to resist false optimism.

April 13, 2024

My 74th birthday. I don't give a damn, nor does anyone else. Bev and Brad are with Shannon. Maybe they took her shopping. I really hope they take her outside! She needs sun, and her kids, and a chocolate shake. She should be having a great day.

April 20, 2024

Brad and Bev were here last weekend. Neither contacted me. Shannon told me that they took her to lunch and shopping. They do very little to camouflage their… what is it… animosity?... resentment?… toward me. We have had our differences, and a few of them concerned me directly. The vast majority of our differences happened because I could not keep my mouth shut… or my keyboard silent… when it came to their mother's care and their unwillingness to shoulder even a little of the financial and physical burden.

Get this. They took her shopping at Target and then took her to lunch at Chipotle, *and they allowed her to pay for lunch.* I saw the charge on her credit card, and, bewildered, asked her about it. Of course, she said that she wanted to do something nice for them after they took her shopping. I was very angry, and she told Brad, who sent me a snippy email volunteering to reimburse me. I replied that I did not want money. I wanted him and Bev to recognize that their mother is dying. I wanted him to shoulder some responsibility. "She is no longer your mother," I told him. "You are now the parent, and I want you to act like it" I wrote.

I KNEW then, as I know now, that each of them will someday realize that they squandered the last opportunities of their lives to spend time with her. The family questions they should be asking her. The sound of her voice. Playing her favorite music. They could be doing that far more often than they have chosen to. I am grateful to them for coming to see Shannon. I am thankful for ANYTHING that gives Shannon a reason to smile. I do not need the assistance that I once did, but I do enjoy seeing Shannon perk up because they visited. Come to think of it, I have not seen her smile in weeks.

April 25, 2024

I go every day to The Blossoms. The staff recognizes me and greets me with smiles. Shannon seems to be doing well, though she complains constantly. I do not blame her for that. I would complain, too. I visit her in the afternoon, and we usually go for a light lunch and a short drive. Much as we did in The Village, but Shannon returns to The Blossoms and I go home alone. The house is lonely without her. I have recaptured all of my lost sleep, and now stay awake until 4 or 5AM involuntarily, but as before, worrying.

May 12, 2024

A terrible thing happened a few days ago. I was preparing to load the Ducati onto the trailer, and I was circling slowly through our cul-de-sac. There is only one other home there. As I executed a U-turn in front of that home, my engine stalled. I was slow getting my foot down and tumbled off of the bike, hitting my head on the pavement. A police car happened to be passing by, and the policeman asked if I needed help. Jean Lewis, our 85-year-old neighbor, peeked out of her front door at that time and asked the same thing. "Yes," I told the policeman. "Yes, Jean…I am bleeding. Could you bring me a wet towel?" As Jean stepped from her home with the towel, I saw that the policeman had left his car in the street and was now sprinting toward her. She had collapsed in her front yard. Within minutes, two more police cars, two ambulances, and a fire truck were on the scene.

One of the policemen pushed the Ducati back to my garage. He found me pouring straight vodka onto my bloody scalp. (I had no alcohol; vodka was my closest alternative.) He said that Jean did not respond. She had died in her front yard of a heart attack (while bringing me a wet towel, he thankfully did not add.) It was Jean's fourth heart attack. Shannon and I had seen the flashing lights of EMS trucks in their driveway twice. Still, I could not escape the thought that I had hastened her death.

May 17, 2024

I am back home after a short trip. My selfishness, needing to just get away for a few days, and my haste in doing so is now impossible for me to explain. Unless there is really such a thing as a man "snapping."

I will see Shannon at noon tomorrow. And begin to make amends.

June 2, 2024

While on the trip, I talked with Shannon every day by phone. She sounded worse on every call. I was, therefore, surprised to find her in good spirits and looking forward to lunch. We went to a BBQ/Korean/Asian fusion restaurant, which she did not like at all, although she tried to be polite about it. That was encouraging. It was, at least, a normal reaction.

I told Shannon about the death of Jean Lewis. Shannon responded, "The old bat already had one foot in the grave."

I had known Shannon for thirteen years, and that was the only mean thing I ever heard her say. This meanness and belligerence are common behaviors in final stage dementia. The change is marked, and important.

June 6, 2024

The Blossoms called me to tell me that Shannon had fallen in her bath and hit her head. They took her to the hospital emergency room to check it out. She is now back in her room and seems to be OK… they say.

June 10, 2024

Bev is in town, and Shannon seems doped. Bev noticed it before me. I might be so accustomed to seeing her decline that my vision is blurred. Or it might have been sudden. But whatever it is, Bev tried to put an end to it, telling the staff to lighten up on the sedatives. I arrived at The Blossoms to find Bev sitting facing Shannon, who was in the common area, slumped forward in her wheelchair. I pulled a chair in front of her and called her name.

Shannon looked straight at me and said, "David Legan!" as if seeing me for the first time in years. She recognized me, but she did not recognize me as her husband. Those were the last words I would hear from Shannon.

June 12, 2024

The nurses at The Blossoms are so concerned about Shannon's stupor that they are transporting her to Baptist Hospital today. There will be more tests. Restricting the drugs, which were thought to be the cause of her state of unconsciousness, did not arouse her. She seems asleep or comatose. She is unresponsive.

June 13, 2024

A nurse within the Palliative Care Unit phoned me this morning before I left my home. I do not remember the purpose of her call, but I DO remember that she said, "You are Shannon's Power of Attorney, so you are my first call…"

I was surprised. Bev should have the Power of Attorney by now, as I had revoked my power upon Bev's request and emailed her a copy of my notarized revocation. Subsequently, I asked Bev if she had followed up and if Shannon had granted HER the power, but she had not. I never heard anything more about it. I thought Bev probably had not found the right time for Shannon to sign.

I did not want to be Shannon's power of attorney. I did not want to be the decider. Very soon, I feared, someone would be forced to decide about Shannon's feeding tube, and I did not want to be that person. I previously told Bev that I felt this way and felt that she and Brad should be responsible for this horrible decision.

Later that day, at the hospital, I met with Bev and Brad. Well, "met" is not really correct – it was no "meeting." It was a deathwatch. We three were sitting silently around Shannon's bed. As Bev stood to leave, I asked, "Bev, can we talk for a minute?"

I began, "There will come a time, probably soon, when you will have to decide… I do not want to make that decision, but I will be watching closely."

Bev was infuriated. She stood up in righteousness and began to lambast me. I simply sat and listened as she shouted at me, "You need to watch the way you say things." (Note: I have been told this before. I am trying to do better.) "You don't need to watch us. You have not even BEEN here most of the time." Sobs were beginning to distort her continuing "lecture." She told me that she met with the palliative folks, and the feeding tube was coming out the next day, and she was going to sit with Shannon for as long as it took, and that is just how it was going to be. And then she ran from the room, still sobbing.

Brad stood and looked at me. I started to say, "That was not really directed at me, Bev is stressed…" but I began sobbing before I could finish. We were all on a razor's edge. After regaining my composure,

I asked Brad if Bev had a Power of Attorney document for Shannon. He did not know, so he phoned Bev to check.

"Yes, she does." Dammit, she never told me.

"If I had known, I'd never have brought it up. Damn. I am not even entitled to an opinion. The nurse called me this morning, and…" my voice trailed off as I realized that my explanation did not matter. The only thing that mattered was Shannon's ever-diminishing breath. It did not matter because I was going to apologize to Bev, thank her for stepping up, and let nature take its course… with her guidance, not mine. It did not matter because, I was convinced, Shannon's death was imminent. No one could help her, and none of us could hurt her. Ever again. It just did not matter.

June 14, 2024

At 11AM, I texted Bev, who was staying with Shannon. "Any news."

"No. She is awake but not alert."

"Well, awake is good." I did not believe that Shannon was awake, or that she would awaken. I gave Bev the benefit of the doubt. Why not allow her to be unrealistically optimistic? Who was I to stand in the way of that?

We were doing that unspeakable service, which families are sometimes called upon to do. Of many family duties, this was the one I dreaded most. There have been other occasions in my life that I have been forced to watch as a comatose person slowly sank toward the inevitable. I thought this to be just like my 18-year-old cousin, struck by a car in his high school parking lot in 1976, like my mom in the ICU in 1996, and like my seven-year-old neighbor, also struck by a car, thirty-five years ago. I could not be certain, of course. But in every case in which I had been a spectator, the comatose patient did not awaken. This was not a movie, there was no heroic doctor breaking down doors with an experimental remedy, and there would be no happy ending.

“Yes, we are going to consult with palliative care today,” texted Bev.

Later that day, she texted, “Probably not a good idea for us to talk on the phone. Are you still at the hospital?”

I returned her text, “Yeah. I’m not angry… you are safe with me.”

June 15, 2024

Brad phoned me this morning and asked if Shannon had signed anything to help with executing her wishes. “A living will?” I asked. “Of course, I have that. I’ll bring it to you.” It was in a three-year-old file. That is how long I had been dealing with an issue that, to him, had suddenly become important that very day.

June 16, 2024

I spent the day with Shannon after arriving at Baptist at 11AM. Her breath seemed steady, and I tried several times to awaken her. “Shannon? Shannon?” No response. Louder, “Shannon, wake up. Shannon, Bev is coming!” Trickery that did not work. Just as it had not worked when I whispered to Aron, my little neighbor, “Aron, wake up… your team needs you!”

Bev texted at 5:30PM, “I was planning to go there around 6:30 unless you wanted to stay longer.” Curious. Did Bev think that I did not want to be around her… that we were still fighting? Or did she simply want to ensure that her mom was not left alone? I did not know, but I was not going to be the person who left Shannon alone.

I texted back, “7 is good. OK with you?”

"Great," she answered. I stayed until she arrived, we exchanged pleasantries, and I departed.

June 17, 2024

Bev ordered the feeding tube removed.

At 11AM, I texted Bev, "Any improvement?"

"A bit. She has more life in her eyes and makes facial expressions. More color on her face. Responding to me, but still no words. Moving arms and legs a lot."

"Sounds like something," I responded, though I silently thought that Bev was looking for something… anything… to hang onto.

June 18, 2024

Shannon's coma continues. I stayed with her until Bev arrived, and it was clear that she was going to spend the night. I should have. I remembered reading that patients like Shannon, old and sick and unconscious, frequently die around 3AM or 4AM. I should have stayed. But I did not.

June 19, 2024

Shannon expired at 4:00AM today. Bev called me at 4:30AM, and I was there at 5:30AM. Bev said that her breath became increasingly shallow until she simply stopped breathing completely.

The nurses came at 6:15 and took my girl away.

Chapter 7
Reflections

When you ask how I've been here without you
I like to say I've been fine, and I do.
John Denver

The caretaking of Shannon did not awaken a hidden genius within me. It did not turn me into Socrates or Twain. I did not gain extraordinary knowledge or wisdom from five years of allowing someone else's needs to preempt my own. As seems often to occur to many authors of self-help manifestos, the writing of a book did not make me smarter or more enlightened than my audience. Shannon and I were remarkably average people. Our exact experiences may have been unique to us, but they were not at all uncommon in a larger sense. In the larger sense, we are all alike.

There are about six million dementia patients in the United States, about one million of those are afflicted with the Lewy Body variant of dementia. The illness of each one affects about five folks within their family or circle of friends. So, in that sense, thirty-five million Americans are suffering from dementia. Each is enduring their own pain.

Each has their own random, shameful thoughts and feels guilty about them. Each is grieving. Every one of them awakens sometimes from tormenting dreams. Each suffers an occasional involuntary shudder when struck by a certain memory. Each is hurting.

A Humble Suggestion

If there is one piece of advice that I can offer to the beginning caretaker, it is this: call for help, NOW. You may not yet be exhausted, but you soon will be. You may not be financially stressed now, but for many of you, that is coming. You may not yet have realized the burden you will be carrying. Before you reach exhaustion or financial stress, ask for help from as many people and sources as you can. In the heat of the coming battle, you will likely not have either time or energy to seek assistance. When you most need help, you may not have the energy to find it. Do everything you can, right now, to NOT be a sole caretaker. I didn't.

Count on the fact that your friends and relatives are unlikely to know the "crush level" of this disease on you. They will not know, specifically, how they can help. They will not know unless you tell them. When communicating with those from whom you might expect assistance, do not believe such promises as, "Just call on me if you need anything. I want to help… ask for anything, anytime." I have found that such promises are seldom kept… they were not meant when offered. "Promises" such as these are usually just conversation fillers… not meant to be taken seriously… just something people say. They are comparable to sending thoughts and prayers to victims of a school shooting. They sound nice but are not often helpful.

So, do not allow those well-meaning folks to get off that easily. Ask for help in specific terms. "Can you take care of Aunt Imogene every Tuesday afternoon while I go grocery shopping?" Or, "Can you contribute $300 each month for respite care?" "Could you arrange for a housekeeper once a week?" Maybe, "Can you take her to her doctor visits twice a month?" Do not be afraid or too proud to tell your circle that you need help. Then offer them specific ways that they can contribute. Soon enough, I can almost promise, you will think of those who should be helping you, but are not, as being hopelessly detached, and you could grow to resent their detachment. The risk here is that this resentment will remain when Aunt Imogene is gone. This burden is hard enough for the time you must carry it. We should try to ensure that there is no remaining burden, after her departure, of damaged relationships. I did not, and it bothers me, still.

You might also investigate community sources of assistance. Adult day care centers. Senior citizens organizations. Volunteers. Support groups. Every municipality has these, so ferret them out. Do not wait to do these things and search for these people later. Later will be too late.

Bless our doctors' hearts. A frequent issue in dealing with Shannon's illness was the lack of guidance from professionals within the medical establishment. They do not want to, or they are not able to deal with specifics of terminal illness. No doctor ever said to me, "Shannon is dying." No physician ever said, "Prepare yourself. You are soon to be alone." I do not resent their reluctance to use the "D word" with patients and loved ones, though I do not understand it, either. So what if doing so is difficult? They signed up for this duty. It is a duty which, if properly satisfied, would benefit each patient and caretaker. And yet, they hedge, obfuscate, and ignore the obvious. Damn, WE KNOW what is happening. Help us!

In this book, I have attempted to address this weakness by revealing what might happen to the next dementia patient, and when, by honestly revealing exactly what happened to us, and when. Dementia Day by Day is not intended to guide or advise. It is not a roadmap. It is only what it presents itself to be: a collection and explanation of dated diary entries that tell the story of two adults who had their lives ended or upended by a terrible disease. This timeline is far more than I was furnished, though I asked for it from every doctor, caregiver, and psychiatrist with whom I spoke.

So, please take these two things from this book. It is a true story, and it is honestly told.

Oh, Dear Diary.

The curse of a diary is that it is written in the present time and only later interpreted. It can be seen in many entries that I was simply wrong. Often unable to make sense of the world I was attempting to navigate. I was wrong frequently, uninformed often, and dozens of times, while assembling this book I was tempted to revise an entry before typing it up for you to read. The entries themselves now reveal my lack of knowledge and understanding. They sometimes reveal my stupidity or propensity to anger quickly. Nevertheless, I resisted that compulsion to revise - in every instance. A revision would steal from the diary its immediacy and honesty. It would be disrespectful of its purpose. I did not write this book to make myself look good, smart, or selfless. This book tells the truth about what Shannon and I were thinking, doing, and experiencing. And when. Warts and all, right here, right now, exposed so that hopefully someone can learn something helpful.

The re-reading of Shannon's Story, the journal itself, was the first time since her death that I confronted death's reality. The reality of hundreds of doctor visits and tearful conversations and scrubbed plans and pain, of exhaustion and stress within the family. Writing Before the Storm, Chapter Two, reminded me of the GOOD years, wherein we formed so many fabulous memories and traveled to such wonderful places. The re-reading of those experiences reminded me of how much we loved and enjoyed one another. That long-ago happiness had been buried in the fog of illness and was only resurrected by attempting to provide her story with context. I am grateful for that, though in bringing back those memories, I found her death even more painful.

Legan's Laws

One: We heal. Healing is the "default position." Absent outside influence, we heal. Our bodies have developed the ability to recover from physical injury. A broken bone takes six weeks. Flesh wounds, about two. Scabs form over cuts, inflammation immobilizes sprained joints, and hypersensitive hearing attempts to replace the loss of eyesight. Mental wounds heal also, though healing time cannot be predicted. (The mind is more complex than skin and bones.) The harm done by stress and sorrow will heal if we only allow ourselves the freedom to heal. It is common, I fear, for folks to hold on to their mental wounds. The damage becomes a self-defining part of the personality. "I hurt, therefore I am."

Expect to heal. Anticipate recovery. Know that you will, indeed that you must, regain strength and continue. That is nature's way. Like it or not, it is our responsibility.

Two: Do it now. Procrastination is the subject of thousands of books and lectures. We all do it, and none of us can explain it, though we know it to be terribly limiting. I am not here to lecture you or sell you another book – you did not buy this book for that. I can state that I recognize it in me, and that I do my best to squash it.

I hold that a thing left unfinished may remain so because we really did not want to do it in the first place. We never committed to it, so we did not do it, and that is just fine!

Far better, however, is that one take stock of this, and say to themselves, "I do not want to do that, and saying so now is better than leaving it on my "to do" list for the next six weeks." THAT is not what we want. Instead, we might commit to not doing it. We might write on our "to-do" list – "Do not return Bill's call," and grin mischieviously every time we see that note. We should make that commitment now. We should decide, rather than leave it to happenstance. That is how we maintain control.

Caretakers and other loved ones should take careful note. This dementia thing. Its vengeful control of your patient's life…it has a tipping point. As the disease builds its strength and saps theirs, as it rampages through their failing bodies, there comes – suddenly – a time when their waning strength has been taxed so much that there is none left. Seemingly overnight, they'll not recognize you. They will not hear you say "I love you. I am going to miss you SO much" the last time. Please do not wait until they no longer know you to say these things. Start too early if you must, say it too often if you must, but do not leave such things unsaid. This sort of regret, I think, is forever.

Three: When one is offered a rare chance, take it. We have all violated, to our ultimate dismay, this rule. When a rare opportunity, or a once-in-a-lifetime experience, or a last chance is presented, be VERY careful about turning it down. Fate is notorious for drafting circumstances to prevent repeat opportunities.

Corollary to Legan's Law Number Three:

Sometimes, we are given only one opportunity to do the right thing. The only way to avoid the danger is to do the right thing every time. Doing the right thing should be a reaction, not a decision.

. . .

Four: Aim high. For your own protection, and the protection of your own self-image, do not consistently underestimate others. Instead, expect friends and associates to do the right thing, to succeed, and to perform admirably. They will not always do so, but it is an act of self-immolation to expect the worst. Aim high, and though one might be frequently disappointed, one is at least not living a life of pessimism.

Five: Expect karma. It's like, you know, when you are just napping, and the world explodes, and it is, like, a serious bummer.

That is what some folks think of when I suggest that their current actions might somehow influence their future. Some folks think of this as a suggestion that a supernatural force is tending to circumstances that influence their lives. That is not the case.

I figure it works like this: good intentions and acts position one to greet a reimbursement of those opportunities and good fortune. It is not the same as saying, "Send good vibes into the universe, and they will come back to you." Rather, it is that those who are kind are likely to recognize kindness when they are treated with kindness. Those who are generous will recognize and appreciate the generosity shown to them. Honest folks will see honesty when treated honestly. Recognition of these acts is only allowed to those who position themselves by their own acts of generosity, kindness, and honesty. Now, this is important; *recognition is everything.* Kindness, generosity, and honesty are mental constructs, and their recognition is their own reward. It is their value, and if they are not recognized, they are nothing.

All grieved out. My grief was surprisingly hollow for the first eight weeks following Shannon's death. I did not begin to grieve "properly" until I began writing this book. I attributed the emptiness in my mind to Shannon's slow and bewildering disease. I had grieved, I reasoned, with every insidious step as her mind left her. With each delusion, I grieved. With each hallucination, I felt what I thought was grief, at that time. But it was not grief. It was disappointment. It was heartbreak. It was relentless sorrow multiplied by stress, resentment, sleeplessness, and, worst of all, hopelessness. There may be a limit to these, beyond which a person cannot step without risking grave psychological harm. I never researched that limit, though I may have approached it.

It appears to me, however, that one's mindset *can* be altered by 24/7 caretaking of a declining loved one. Such an alteration might manifest, even to the caretaker, as a tepid reaction to the death of the loved one. Or worse, it might make the caretaker feel even more guilty, amplifying their sorrow with self-doubt and flagellation.

"What? No grief?"

"I must have spent all of my available grief a little at a time, and now I am all grieved out."

Bullshit is what that is. The grief is there. It is locked up with other emotions that have been suppressed for years. It is hiding, awaiting the perfect time to ambush. It will come, raging into your heart, in its own time; and it will be more vicious, more disabling, more wrenching than you imagined possible. Mine was. Still is.

No one should denigrate themselves for feeling less than appropriately morose. One who has made caregiver levels of sacrifice should not think of themselves as heartless. We build fences around our hearts, and those fences are part of a self-defense system that developed within us naturally, as common a reaction as a wince to a pinprick. We avoid pain, and when we cannot avoid it, like an oyster, we cover it in crust.

One thousand days of service.

I have spoken with many survivor-caretakers. Each of them thinks of their service as the most impactful event of their lives. Each is proud of their work. Each is crushed by their loss. Each will carry that pride and loss to their graves. Unsurprisingly, each feels somewhat guilty. Guilty over… what? That they did not do enough? That they, themselves, were spared? That they do not deserve the good fortune of continuing to exist? You see the irrationality of these thoughts, yet you intuitively understand. You nod in agreement. You know.

The caretaking of a hopelessly terminal patient is a burden. Caretakers cannot run from that. There are steps that a caretaker can take to protect themselves from the physical harm that comes from carrying such a heavy emotional weight. Many of you have heard or read this, as did I. Like me, many of you will not heed those warnings. I get that.

"I am different!" "I can handle it!" "It's no burden… it is love," one tells oneself. Again, bullshit. Most folks do not, as I did not, understand the weight of the burden before shouldering it. We see that we are needed, and we step up. In that moment we make a decision that will shape our lives for years at least and very likely for the remainder of our days. That may be, in its purest form, society's principal defense against the weight of six million dementia patients. We may be guided by invisible forces to ignore the burden we place on ourselves, and the harm it can cause, for the greater good.

How else could the patient receive the one-on-one care they need without the tendency of caretakers to give too much and care too much and suffer disproportionatly? Could it be that we, as a species, have evolved these self-sacrificing behaviors because our society benefits? Could there be an invisible community conscience that guides us to make incredible sacrifices for those we do not even know, by taking care of those we love?

The renowned archeologist Margaret Mead was once asked, "Which of your discoveries was the earliest sign of civilization?" Was it cave drawings or pottery or tools? None of those. It was the femur of an old man which had been broken – and been allowed time to heal. Someone took care of the old man for weeks as his leg healed. He was not abandoned. He was housed and fed, accompanied, and transported while he was unable to care for himself. THAT is civilization. As cave dwellers, individuals contributed with physical goods. They brought food to the cave. They fought intruders, skinned hides, and gathered fruit. But it was when they began to care for one another that they became civilized. Without caretakers, we are only a step away from the caves. Maybe there is truth in that.

You may decide this for yourself. Beyond baring my heart to you in this book, I cannot help, and I am finished.

Epilogue

Thank You, I'm Sorry

Don't confront me with my failures, I had not forgotten them.
Jackson Browne

Thanks and heartfelt appreciation to:
Claude Mahend
Dr. Hillary Williams, and her supporting staff at University of Arkansas Medical School

I promised not to edit the diary. Re-reading the diary forced me to again rethink that promise. I realized that each diary entry was comprised of whatever was "top of mind" that day, and therefore not random. If something angered me or broke my heart that day, then it would likely be mentioned. If I had waited even a day to write, whatever it was that hurt me yesterday might not have made the cut. Oh, I'll not back off of a single word, it is true as it happened. I do wish that my entries had been kinder to Bev and Brad. Like I was, they were dealing with Shannon's impending death for the first time. But they were clueless, and I was not. I had watched my parents die hospital-bound long-suffering deaths; though I did not know when

Shannon's life would end, I did know how. I knew that time would drag out and slow down until, may I be damned for saying it out loud, some would think, "Wouldn't she be better off if her suffering ended… if she died." I knew there would come a time when a bitter sweetness would replace the grief and exhaustion. Most importantly, I knew there were things that simply had to be done "before" because there would be no "after." They were not old enough to know these things, and they were not humble enough to listen to me.

So, Bev and Brad, I am sorry that I wrote hurtful things about you when you hurt me. I am old enough to know better.

Bev, thank you for arranging Shannon's memorial last August tenth. Shannon would have approved of it and the tavern in which it was held, and all of the proceedings. Thanks to my progeny, Macy, Hank and David for attending and holding my hand.

As I write these final words in December 2024, I am beginning to heal. Still untethered, still floating like a balloon in the Superdome, but no longer *hopelessly* doing so. The lawsuit is still in the courts, but a trial date HAS been set. Cricket, despite not seeming to like me very much, is MY friend and sleeping partner. She stalks the hall in the early morning hours and moans as if searching for Buddy… or maybe Shannon.

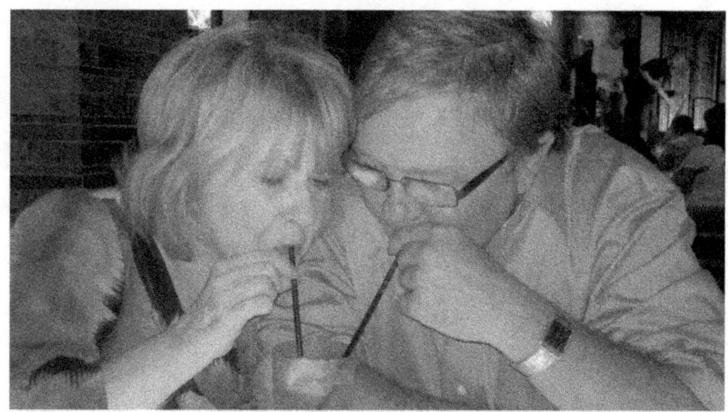

2011, First date

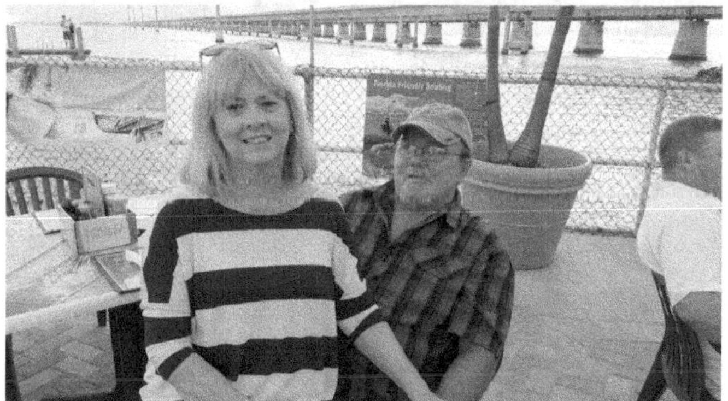

Key West, 2015

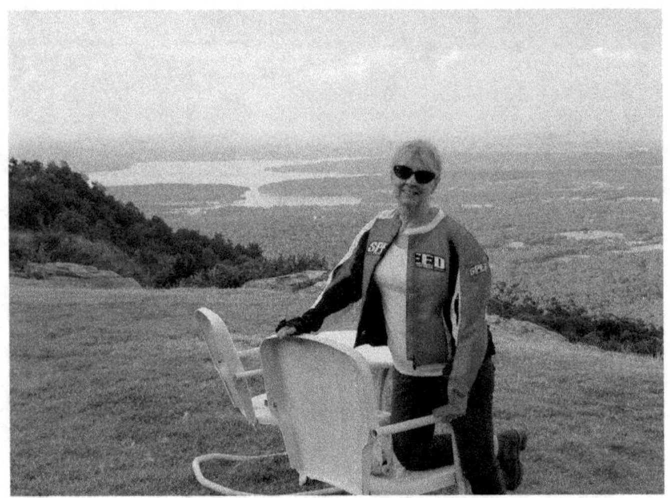

2016 at Sunset Point, The Ozarks

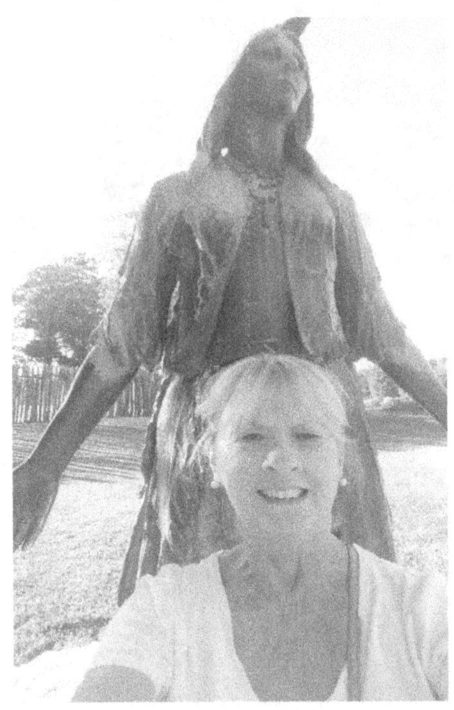

Washington, DC 2016

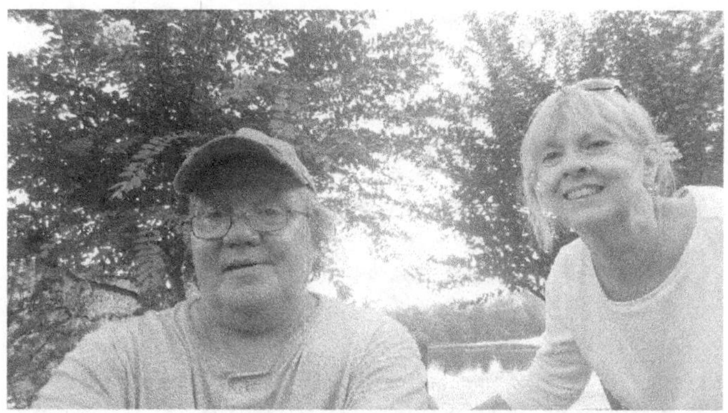

2016, Just after moving to Hot Springs Village

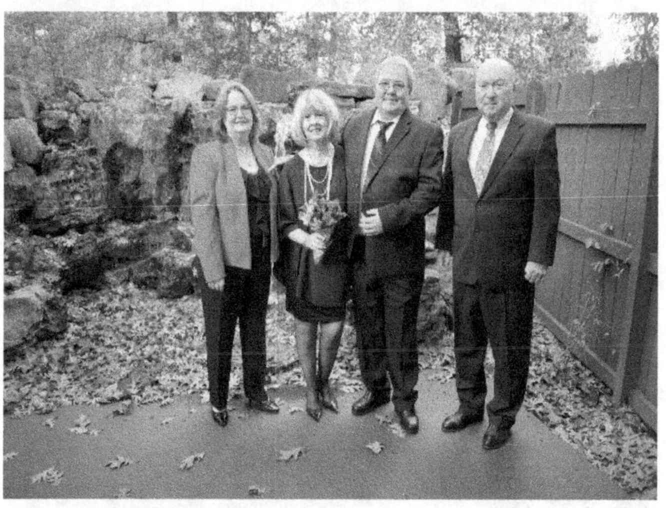

2018, our wedding, with Patricia and Gary Hayes

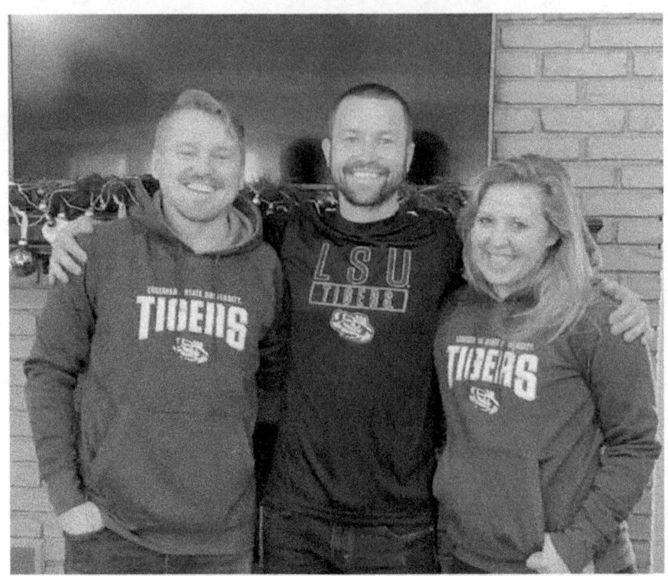

My three, David, Hank, Macy 2019

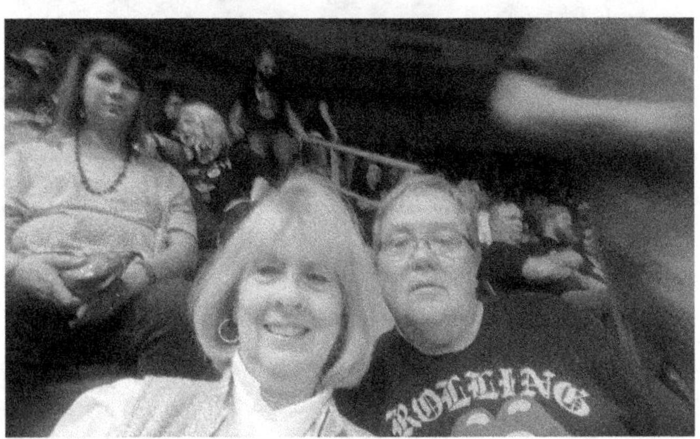

Paul McCartney Concert, 2020

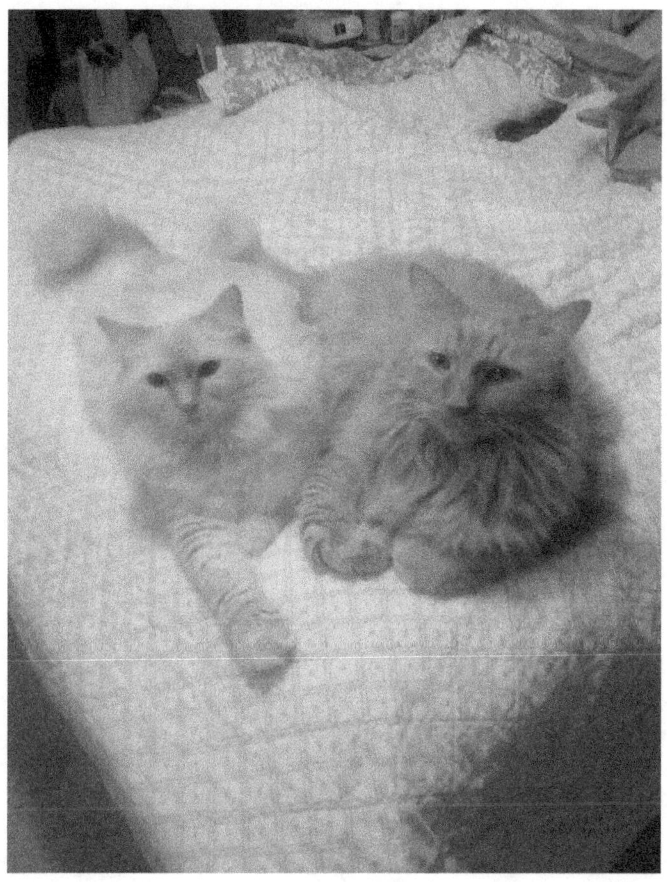

Cricket and Buddy, 2021

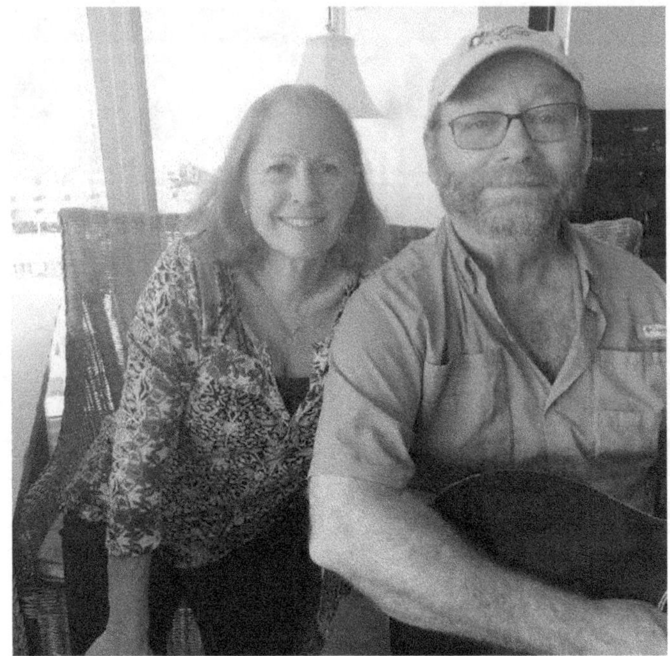

Kathy and Charlie Grau, 2022

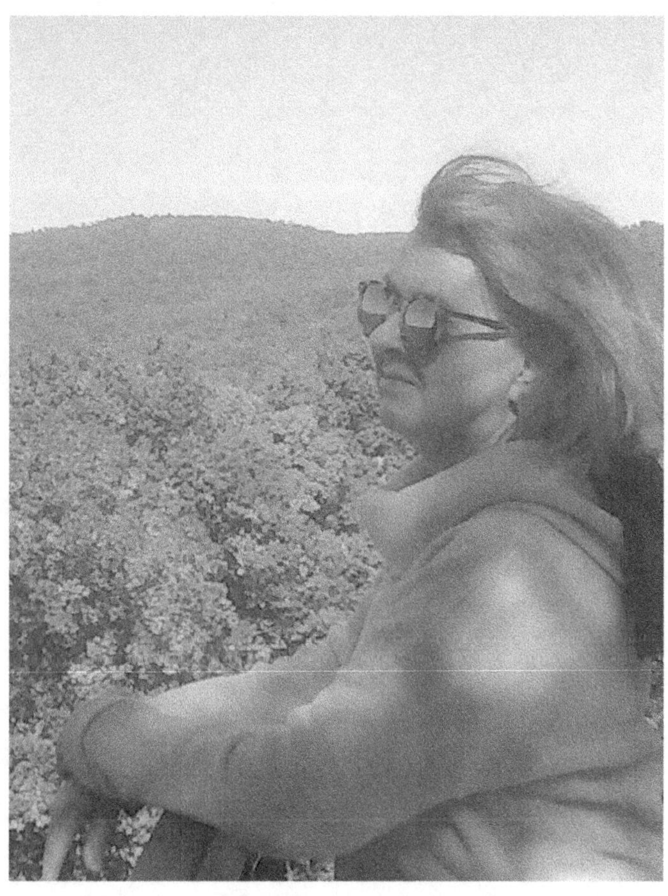

Wedding Weekend, 2018

www.ingramcontent.com/pod-product-compliance
Lightning Source LLC
LaVergne TN
LVHW010555160826
845677LV00013B/3142

* 9 7 9 8 8 9 5 6 9 9 6 2 1 *